Standards

for Obstetric-Gynecologic Services

Sixth Edition

The American College of
Obstetricians and Gynecologists

The Sixth Edition of *Standards for Obstetric-Gynecologic Services* has been developed by the 1982-85 Committee on Professional Standards. The committee wishes to express appreciation to the Committee on Obstetrics: Maternal and Fetal Medicine, the Committee on Gynecologic Practice, the Health Care Commission, and the Executive Board for their review and helpful comments.

1982-85 COMMITTEE ON PROFESSIONAL STANDARDS

Chairman Richard M. Hebertson, MD

Members Philip A. Corfman, MD
Van R. Jenkins, MD
Henry Jacob Koch, MD
Ganson Purcell, MD
Richard W. Stander, MD
Susan M. Tucker, RN

Staff Ervin E. Nichols, MD, Director-Practice Activities
Shirley A. Shelton, Associate Director-Practice Activities
Rebecca D. Rinehart, Editor
R. Michael Dodd, Art Director

It is important, particularly to those agencies or individuals who may consult this manual in preparing codes and regulations governing the delivery of obstetric-gynecologic health care, to recognize that the standards set forth here are presented as recommendations and general guidelines rather than as a body of rigid rules. They are intended to be adapted to many different situations, taking into account the needs and resources particular to the locality, the institution, or type of practice. Variations and innovations that demonstrably improve the quality of patient care are to be encouraged rather than restricted.

Contents

4 Gynecology: Ambulatory Care 51

5 Gynecology: Hospital Care

6 Special Considerations

Preface

Advances in medical knowledge and the way in which such knowledge is applied in health care delivery systems are constantly evolving. This dictates not only the evaluation of routine practices but also assessment in light of cost/benefit ratios at a time when attention is focused on controlling health care expenditures, fostering competition, and implementing cost management measures. To keep pace, guidelines that ensure the quality of care and at the same time take into consideration the need to balance quality with cost/benefit must be subject to a consistent degree of scrutiny and revision.

Such is the case with the sixth edition of *Standards for Obstetric-Gynecologic Services*, which has been in development over the past three years. As a part of the College's commitment to define broadly what constitutes current acceptable standards for the health care of women, these recommendations have been, and will continue to be, reevaluated on an on-going basis.

This process, coordinated by the Committee of Professional Standards, culminates in a consensus of the numerous ACOG committees and medical authorities who lend their expertise to its development. Such a broad scope, reflecting current practice standards as well as ACOG policies and recommendations, is essential to achieve guidelines that can serve as a foundation for the application of basic principles in a variety of settings. The assistance of the many individuals of special competence who collaborated in the development of *Standards of Obstetric-Gynecologic Services* is recognized with gratitude.

As a result of this collaborative effort, new information has been included and refinements have been incorporated in the existing text. For the first time, minimum requirements for obstetric facilities have been outlined and guidelines have been given for the prophylactic administration of Rh immune globulin and glucose screening. The chapters have been reorganized for ease of reference, and standardized definitions have been added to promote consistency in terminology. The discussion of professional privileges has been revised and complemented with an example of how a system based on category of privileges can be implemented. Guidelines for monitoring patients in the delivery room when electronic fetal monitoring was used during labor have been added, and criteria for the early discharge of obstetric patients outlined.

Standards for Obstetric-Gynecologic Care are intended to provide an appropriate balance that assures quality of care is not endangered as increasing attention is focused on rising medical costs. In order to fulfill this function, these standards must be interpreted broadly and not considered hard and fast rules. Flexible, innovative approaches to patient care, based on individual circumstances, are an essential element of the practice of obstetrics and gynecology—the foundation for the health of future generations.

Introduction

The specialty of obstetrics and gynecology is devoted to the health care of women. It encompasses both normal and abnormal processes of the reproductive system of women, including the medical and surgical management of disorders, pregnancy and childbirth, and primary and preventive medical care. The obstetrician-gynecologist, by virtue of special education, training, and skills, is equipped to meet the diverse health care needs of women and to provide continuity of care.

The obstetrician-gynecologist is often a woman's principal source of medical care and, in some instances, her only regular medical contact. In this role, the obstetrician-gynecologist can reinforce good health habits such as regular breast examinations, periodic cervical cytology sampling, family planning and preconceptional counseling, nutrition, and exercise. With strong emphasis on prenatal care and childbirth education and with promotion of a family-centered approach to maternity care, the obstetrician-gynecologist can play a major role in making the childbirth experience safer and more meaningful.

In gynecologic surgery, as in any surgical specialty, skill in diagnosis, knowledge of the natural history and pathophysiology of the disease process, awareness of alternative medical and surgical treatments, and familiarity with the problems of immediate postoperative care and long-term follow-up are as important as surgical skill. The surgeon who performs gynecologic surgery should be familiar with medical gynecology and with the possible effects of pregnancy on other physiologic processes. The obstetrician-gynecologist is best qualified to fulfill these criteria. Accordingly, where qualified obstetrician-gynecologists are available, it should be established policy that these physicians manage complications of pregnancy and perform gynecologic operations.

Some obstetrician-gynecologists have acquired additional special skills or training related to the management of gynecologic malignancies, problems of reproductive dysfunction, and specific high-risk conditions of pregnancy. In addition to certifying physicians in obstetrics and gynecology, the American Board of Obstetrics and Gynecology certifies special competence in the subspecialties of maternal and fetal medicine, gynecologic oncology, and reproductive endocrinology.

In some circumstances, the obstetrician-gynecologist may serve solely as a consultant. In these instances, the patient should be made aware of the need for and scope of care provided and, if necessary, offered assistance in locating a physician to be responsible for her continuing care.

The role of the obstetrician-gynecologist includes broad emphasis on women's health care in general and disorders of the female reproductive system in particular. Providing such care involves specialized skills and training, awareness of a woman's overall health problems, and interaction with health care professionals both within and outside the specialty. It is the responsibility of the obstetrician-gynecologist to monitor patient management, to direct the efforts of the health care team, and to ensure that high-quality care is provided.

These are the goals to which the discipline is dedicated. By continuously evaluating and upgrading the standard of care, as outlined in the following guidelines, the goals of the specialty can be translated into practices that promote women's health.

1
Organization

Quality obstetric-gynecologic care requires efficient organization of the medical staff and other personnel, whether the care is provided within an ambulatory or a hospital setting.

AMBULATORY CARE

Ambulatory obstetric-gynecologic care may be provided in a physician's office, outpatient clinic, or freestanding or hospital-based surgical facility. The organization of the ambulatory care facility varies, depending on the kind of facility or type of practice and on the patient volume. Certain standards are applicable to all types of settings, however.

Personnel directly involved in the welfare of obstetric and gynecologic patients should be organized into a health care team under the direction of an obstetrician-gynecologist. A sufficient number of staff members should be available to prevent undue delays, and they should possess the appropriate skills to provide optimal care. Job descriptions and written policies should be prepared and reviewed periodically. These policies should indicate specific responsibilities, as well as a plan for continuing education of personnel.

A freestanding ambulatory surgical facility should have a governing body, similar to a hospital board of trustees, that has final authority and responsibility for patient care, facilities, services, appointment of the medical staff, and delineation of clinical privileges. A mechanism similar to that used in the hospital for granting privileges should be established. Privileges granted to a physician should not exceed those held by that physician in at least one accredited hospital within the geographic area. A hospital-based facility usually functions under the hospital's governing body, and staff privileges in such a facility are established by hospital regulations.

Details on the way in which a freestanding or hospital-based ambulatory facility should be organized and the relation of the hospital staff to the facility are available from the Joint Commission on Accreditation of Hospitals and the Accreditation Association for Ambulatory Health Care, Inc.

HOSPITAL CARE

RESPONSIBILITY AND AUTHORITY

Ultimate responsibility for patient care, staff, facilities, and services resides in the governing body of the hospital. This body customarily delegates administrative responsibility to an administrator and medical responsibility to the medical staff. The hospital's governing body should establish guidelines to ensure cooperation between these two groups.

The responsibility of departments or sections of the medical staff should be established by the staff and approved by the hospital's governing body. As a discipline, obstetrics and gynecology should be organized as an independent department. The lines of authority within the department should be clearly delineated and must be respected by individuals to whom privileges are granted.

DEPARTMENT ORGANIZATION

The type of organization appropriate for a department of obstetrics and gynecology is determined by the size and type of hospital and by the bylaws of the medical staff. The organizational needs of a hospital devoted exclusively to patient care may differ from those of a hospital with teaching and research responsibilities. There are, however, principles and objectives common to all hospital departments. The following general guidelines should be adapted to local need and custom.

Officers

The staff of the department of obstetrics and gynecology should be directed by a department head, who may be either elected or appointed. The choice of a department head should be based on professional ability, experience, and interest in departmental activities rather than on popularity, size of practice, or seniority on the staff. The practice of rotating the position among all attending staff members is particularly discouraged. The term of office should be at least 3 years to allow the department head adequate time to plan and develop departmental activities. If the department head is appointed and the term of office is more than 5 years, provision should be made for periodic review of the appointment by a designated body, usually a joint conference committee composed of persons selected from the medical staff and governing board.

The department head's responsibilities should be clearly defined by both the medical staff and the hospital administration. The extent of the department head's responsibility should be indicated, at least in broad outline, in the medical staff bylaws. Among the duties of the position, a department head may be expected to assume the following responsibilities:

- Represent the department on the medical staff executive committee
- Formulate a mechanism to maintain adequate continuing medical education for department members
- Submit recommendations on the appointment, reappointment, promotion, or suspension of all department staff physicians
- Evaluate and document periodically the professional performance of each member of the department staff
- Submit recommendations on the granting or withdrawal of privileges in obstetrics and gynecology for members of the department and for members of other departments who request such privileges
- Collaborate with the nursing department in establishing and monitoring policies and procedures for patient care
- Establish the teaching and patient care responsibilities of all staff physicians and prepare a schedule of assignments
- Appoint members to appropriate department committees
- Recommend members of the department for appointment to hospital committees
- Serve as consultant or arbitrator for unresolved differences of opinion in questions of policy
- Make recommendations regarding the obstetric and gynecologic care of patients in other services
- Be responsible for resident and student educational programs

The proper operation of a department of obstetrics and gynecology depends on the cooperation of its members, whose opinions should be obtained concerning major matters of policy. When making decisions that affect other clinical departments and supporting services, the department head should consult with the heads of the departments affected.

It is often advisable to elect or appoint a secretary. Written minutes of department meetings are essential, both to provide continuity in the activities of the department and to keep the medical staff and administration informed.

If a department staff fund is maintained, it is recommended that one or more members share the control of this fund with the department head. Such an arrangement is particularly desirable when contributions to the fund come from the efforts of staff members. Accurate records should be kept, and a periodic audit should be performed. A treasurer, who may be elected or appointed, or a department advisory committee may be responsible for overseeing such a fund.

Committees

Members of the department are expected to participate in the work of the department. Because involvement encourages interest, staff members should be given specific responsibilities in the department or assigned to committees. Committee activities should include assessments of the quality of care by reviewing maternal and perinatal deaths; significant maternal, perinatal, and gynecologic morbidity; and resource utilization. These reviews can identify potential problems for further evaluation.

In departments with a large number of staff members, an executive or advisory committee is desirable to expedite the decision-making process and to provide for staff representation. When the staff has several components, such as full-time, part-time, or volunteer personnel, each component should be represented on the committee.

Membership

Depending on the size and organization of the hospital, the staff members of the department may include, in addition to obstetrician-gynecologists, other physicians with a special interest in obstetrics and gynecology. Membership and rank should be contingent on not only fulfillment of the qualifications established by the hospital, but also a willingness to support the department's policies and to contribute to its activities.

PROFESSIONAL PRIVILEGES

To maintain high standards of care and service, it is necessary to ensure that each physician provides only those services for which he or she is qualified by training and experience. The degree of complexity and specificity required for the delineation of professional privileges is determined by the size of the hospital and the services and skills available. Privileges should be defined in a way that ensures quality of care to each patient, meets the needs of the community, fulfills the hospital's responsibility to its staff and governing board, applies criteria fairly and uniformly, and provides due process. Privileges should be granted on the basis of education, experience, and demonstrated competence, not solely on the basis of board certification, fellowship in the American College of Obstetricians and Gynecologists, membership in other scientific organizations, or the physician's rank or tenure. It is the responsibility of each service or department to recommend to the appropriate committee of the medical staff a method of delineating privileges, and this method must subsequently be approved by the hospital governing body.

An initial appointment to the medical staff should be based on a thorough review of the individual's credentials. The appointment should include a designated classification of privileges and a provisional period of established duration (usually 6 months to 1 year). Staff bylaws may provide for an extension of the provisional period if the volume of work or the opportunity for observation has not been sufficient to satisfy the requirements for regular staff eligibility. An appointee found to be professionally competent and ethical at the end of the provisional interval should be granted regular staff membership with an appropriate classification of privileges. If, at the end of the provisional time, there is documented evidence that the individual has not demonstrated professional competence, it should be recommended to the hospital's governing body that privileges be restricted or terminated. Any such action should be subject to the procedural rights established in the local medical staff bylaws.

A nonspecialist may acquire sufficient knowledge and experience to warrant an extension of specified privileges in obstetrics and gynecology. The granting of such privileges to a member of another clinical department should be initially recommended by that department and then approved by the department of obstetrics and gynecology.

Classifications

There are three common methods of classification of professional privileges: 1) designation by illnesses, conditions, injuries, and procedures; 2) designation by specialties; or 3) categorical designation.

Designation by comprehensive lists is cumbersome and unnecessarily detailed, and designation by specialties alone may be inappropriate in that it does not take into consideration the amount, or lack, of experience a physician may have. The latter method also fails to identify staff members who have voluntarily restricted their own practices.

Delineation of privileges by category is preferable to other methods (Table 1–1). Illnesses, conditions, and procedures are grouped into categories that reflect progressive degrees of patient care complexity, of risk to the patient, and of training and experience that the physician needs to

Table 1-1. Delineation of Professional Privileges by Category

CATE-GORY	DEGREE OF COMPLEXITY AND/OR RISK TO PATIENT	QUALIFICATIONS	OBSTETRIC EXAMPLES	GYNECOLOGIC EXAMPLES
I	Diagnosis and therapy with minimal threat to life	Physician with minimal formal training in the discipline but with training and experience in the care of specific conditions	Normal antepartum and postpartum care Uncomplicated labor and delivery Maternal-fetal monitoring Administration of local anesthesia and pudendal block Episiotomy and repair of second degree laceration Use of oxytocic drugs after completion of third stage of labor	Assistance in gynecologic surgery
II	Major diagnosis and therapy but with no significant threat to life	Physician with significant graduate training in the specialty related to diagnosis and therapy; i.e. • full ___ months of training and experience in approved obstetric training program • full ___ months of training and experience in approved gynecologic training program • experience in the care of specific conditions	Category I Amniotomy Manual rotations Elective low forceps Manual removal of placenta and postpartum uterine exploration Repair of third degree perineal laceration Circumcision of newborn male	Category I Minor gynecologic surgery

III	Major diagnosis and therapy with possible serious threat to life	Physician with completed residency training in the specialty or with extensive training or experience in the care of specific conditions	Categories I and II All vaginal deliveries All cesarean deliveries All high-risk pregnancies including major medical diseases complicating pregnancy except intra-uterine transfusions	Categories I and II All gynecologic illnesses and complications All gynecologic procedures except: Radical vulvectomy Radical hysterectomy Pelvic exenteration Pelvic radiation therapy Microsurgery Laser surgery
IV	Unusually complex or critical diagnosis and therapy with possible serious threat to life	Physician with significant formal training beyond completion of residency requirements related to diagnosis or therapy (acquisition of additional privileges related to new technologies should be based on appropriate formal education, experience, and performance under observation)	Categories I, II, and III Intrauterine transfusions	Categories I, II, and III Specific privileges: Radical vulvectomy Radical hysterectomy Pelvic exenteration Pelvic radiation therapy Microsurgery Laser surgery

manage them. Department members establish written guidelines that delineate which illnesses, conditions, and procedures are in each category. Categories may vary with the size of the hospital and the services it provides. An appropriate category is assigned to each physician. Illnesses, conditions, and procedures that fall within another category may be added to a physician's category of privileges when it has been determined that the physician is qualified to manage them. Those staff members with a high category of privileges are usually entitled to privileges of the lower categories unless otherwise indicated. The various categories can range from I through IV.

Regardless of the method used for the delineation of privileges, each department or hospital staff should establish its own specific regulations according to local need and professional resources available.

Reevaluation

The clinical competence of each staff member should be documented continually. The department should systematically reevaluate, at least every 2 years, each member's clinical privileges, using information from the individual member's file. This file should contain evidence of medical education, continuing medical education, professional recognition, results of various methods of quality care evaluation, and professional sanction, if any. Following examination of the file, recommendations should be made to the governing body of the hospital as to whether privileges should remain unchanged or should be expanded, restricted, or terminated. If privileges are to be restricted or terminated, the staff member should be given the recommendations and the basis for them in writing. Review before the appropriate hospital staff committees should be guaranteed to staff members when questions concerning restrictions or terminations of privileges arise. Final action and authority reside with the governing body. Formal review of the proceedings by this body should be available to the staff member with provision made for another formal review if requested.

Emergency Care

Provision should be made in hospital bylaws for emergency medical care. The bylaws should authorize members of the medical staff, in an emergency, to treat any medical disease or perform surgical procedures at the hospital if delay in administering treatment may result in serious harm to, or be an immediate threat to the life of, the patient.

Nonphysician Personnel

When licensed by the state, personnel other than physicians, including nurse-practitioners, certified nurse-midwives, and physician-assistants, may provide health care under the direction of a physician. Specific delineation of privileges for the care provided by these personnel should be written and approved by the department of obstetrics and gynecology, the appropriate committee of the medical staff, and the governing body of the hospital.

2
Obstetrics: Ambulatory Care

Every woman should have a comprehensive program of obstetric care that begins as early as possible in the first trimester of pregnancy, and preferably before conception, and extends through the postpartum period. Early diagnosis of pregnancy and risk assessment are important to establish the management plan appropriate to the individual. The concept of family-centered care, emphasizing family involvement in the childbirth experience, is an important aspect of obstetrics. Consideration of each patient's special needs—medical, emotional, and educational—can help promote quality obstetric care.

SERVICES

The physician and other members of the health care team should discuss the proposed plan of obstetric care with the patient. The discussion should include an explanation of office care; necessary laboratory studies; expected course of the pregnancy; signs and symptoms to be reported to the physician; timing of subsequent office visits; educational programs; alternative birthing procedures; and the general plan for hospital admission, labor, delivery and postpartum care. The discussion should also include an explanation of the roles of various members of the health care team, office policies (including how to reach the physician in an emergency), and alternate physician coverage. Specific information regarding costs should be provided so that the patient can make financial arrangements for care.

ANTEPARTUM CARE

Initial and periodic evaluation of the patient's status and special attention to risk factors are key aspects of antepartum care. In addition to monitoring the pregnancy, this is a good time for the physician to provide education and positive reinforcement to the patient in matters relating to health and childbirth.

Initial Evaluation

During the initial evaluation, an obstetric data base should be established for each patient. It should include a comprehensive health history with information on the current pregnancy, family and social history, a physical examination, laboratory procedures, and risk assessment.

The health history should include menstrual history, methods of family planning, and a detailed record of the current and past pregnancies and data that allow the physician to estimate the date of delivery. Information on the current pregnancy should include factors that help identify the patient at high risk. Such factors include age, vaginal bleeding, edema, urinary infection, rubella, exposure to radiation and chemicals, ingestion of certain drugs and alcohol, and use of tobacco. The past obstetric review should include the number of full-term pregnancies, premature deliveries, and spontaneous and induced abortions; the number of living children; spacing of previous pregnancies; length of each gestation; route of delivery; sex and weight of the newborn; and any complications, particularly those resulting in fetal or neonatal deaths.

Emphasis should be placed on drug sensitivities and other allergies, operations, blood transfusions, blood group and Rh type, diabetes and other metabolic diseases, vascular problems, sexually transmitted diseases, convulsive disorders, gynecologic abnormalities, and serious injuries. The previous administration of Rh immune globulin should be noted specifically.

The family history should include information on metabolic disorders, cardiovascular disease, malignancy, congenital abnormalities, mental retardation, and multiple births. The social history should include the patient's occupation and work environment, ethnic origin, and educational background. Religious beliefs precluding or mandating certain types of therapy should be noted.

A comprehensive physical examination should be performed during the initial prenatal evaluation. This should include an evaluation of nutritional status, height, weight, and blood pressure, as well as examination of the head, neck, breasts, heart, lungs, abdomen, pelvis, rectum, and extremities. During the pelvic examination, attention should be given to the size of the uterus in relation to the presumed duration of the pregnancy, and to the configuration and capacity of the bony pelvis.

The following prenatal laboratory tests should be performed as early in each pregnancy as possible:

- Hemoglobin or hematocrit measurement
- Urinalysis
- Blood group and Rh type determination
- Antibody screen
- Rubella antibody titer measurement
- Syphilis screen
- Cervical cytology

The need for additional laboratory evaluations is determined by pertinent findings derived from the history and physical examination. These may include urine culture, determination of blood glucose level, culture for gonorrhea, examination for sickle cell and other inheritable diseases, and tuberculosis skin testing.

Based on the findings of the history and physical exam, a risk assessment should be determined indicating risk factors that may require special management. Such factors could include:

- Cesarean delivery, including type of uterine incision
- Operations on the uterus or cervix
- Medical indication for termination of pregnancy
- Premature onset of labor
- History of prolonged labor suggesting dystocia
- Two or more abortions, spontaneous or induced
- Newborn small or large for gestational age
- Multiple gestation
- Neonatal morbidity
- Fetal or neonatal death
- Isoimmunization
- Cardiovascular disease
- Urinary tract disorders
- Metabolic or endocrine disease
- Chronic pulmonary disease
- Nutritional disorder
- Maternal use of drugs, alcohol, and tobacco
- Maternal age less than 15 years or more than 35 years
- Previous infertility
- Neurologic disorder
- Psychologic illness
- Congenital abnormalities
- Sexually transmitted disease

Recommendations for the management of any problem should be formulated. The risk factors should be reevaluated throughout the pregnancy. The obstetrician should keep the pediatrician apprised of those risk factors that may have a significant bearing on the fetus.

Subsequent Care

The frequency of return visits should be determined by the woman's individual needs and risk assessment. While some degree of flexibility is desirable, the woman with an uncomplicated pregnancy should generally be seen every 4 weeks for the first 28 weeks of pregnancy, every 2 to 3 weeks until 36 weeks of gestation, and weekly thereafter. Women with active medical or obstetric problems should be seen more frequently, at intervals to be determined by the nature and severity of the problems.

At each follow-up visit the patient should be given an opportunity to ask questions about her pregnancy and to comment on changes she has perceived since the last visit. The physical examination should include blood pressure, weight, measured fundal height, fetal presentation, and fetal heart rate. A urinalysis for protein and sugar should be performed during each visit. Any change in pregnancy risk should be recorded.

Early in the third trimester, the hemoglobin or hematocrit level should be determined again. Since maternal age is a risk factor for diabetes, it is recommended that glucose screening should be performed on women at least by 30 years of age or older. Repeat tests for sexually transmitted diseases should be performed if the patient belongs to a high-risk population. At some time during the patient's antepartum course, it may be appropriate to repeat an antibody screen. An unsensitized Rho(D) negative patient should have a repeat antibody test at about 28 weeks of gestation. If the patient is still unsensitized, she should receive Rh immune globulin prophylactically.

Plans for hospital admission, labor, and delivery should be reviewed and information provided on what to do when labor begins, when the membranes rupture, or when bleeding occurs. Analgesic and anesthetic options should be discussed. Because a general anesthetic may be required for labor and delivery, the patient should be advised of the hazards of ingesting food or fluid after the onset of labor.

Various forms of biochemical or biophysical monitoring may be required to determine the integrity of the fetoplacental unit in high-risk patients. These evaluations may be conducted on an outpatient basis. If amniocentesis is performed, ultrasound should be used to locate the placenta, and the fetal heart rate should be monitored. When amniocentesis is performed in the third trimester, facilities for cesarean delivery should be readily available. Amniocentesis should be performed only by a physician specially trained in the procedure. Unsensitized Rho(D) negative women who undergo amniocentesis should receive Rh immune globulin prophylactically. The amniotic fluid need not be tested in the hospital's laboratory; however, in order to be clinically useful, the results should be available within 24 hours.

Genetic Disorders

Antenatal screening for genetic disorders is an integral part of obstetric care. In some instances, identification of possible risks and appropriate diagnostic measures can be undertaken prior to pregnancy.

The history obtained during the initial evaluation should be reviewed to detect signs of possible genetic disorders: abnormal outcome of a previous pregnancy, family history of birth defects, mental retardation, and other known or suspected inherited or metabolic disorders. Couples who have increased risks for producing abnormal offspring may undergo antenatal diagnostic studies after appropriate counseling. The following factors are indicative of such risk:

- Advanced maternal age (35 years or older at expected time of delivery)
- Previous offspring with a chromosomal aberration, particularly autosomal trisomy
- Chromosomal abnormality in either parent, particularly a translocation
- Family history of a sex-linked condition
- Inborn errors of metabolism
- Neural tube defects
- Hemoglobinopathies

Amniocentesis, fetoscopy, chorionic villus sampling, ultrasound examination, and cytogenetic assessment are some of the tests used for antenatal genetic diagnosis. Physicians should not hesitate to seek consultations with specialists in the antenatal diagnosis of genetic disorders.

HEALTH PROMOTION AND MAINTENANCE

The patient's lifestyle and attitude can have a bearing on her pregnancy and subsequent resumption of normal activities. The obstetrician can take advantage of the doctor-patient relationship established during prenatal care to detect potentially harmful influences and to reinforce positive behavior both during pregnancy and afterward.

Nutrition

The patient's nutritional status and habits should be evaluated during the initial visit and monitored throughout pregnancy, particularly in relation to smoking, alcohol use, or the ingestion of other drugs. Special attention should be given to the dietary habits of the adolescent who is pregnant.

Pregnant women generally require approximately 15% more kilocalories than nonpregnant women. Pregnant women need approximately 150 more kcal/day during the first trimester and 350 kcal/day more during each of the last two trimesters. Thus, an average increase of 300 kcal/day is usual. Protein, iron, folic acid, and certain other vitamins and minerals are required in greater amounts during pregnancy. If these needs are not met by increased dietary intake, a vitamin/mineral supplement equal to the Recommended Dietary Allowances (RDA) for pregnant women should be given.

Nursing mothers need approximately 500 kcal/day more than non-pregnant women. Calcium and protein are also required in increased amounts.

Weight gain should not be rigidly restricted; a total gain of 10-12 kg (22-27 lb) is generally acceptable. Weight reduction during pregnancy is not recommended and may in fact be harmful to the developing fetus. Also, sodium restriction is not usually necessary.

Health and Childbirth Education

The patient is ultimately responsible for her own behavior, and the health care team should provide her with information on which to base critical decisions concerning her health. Such information should be adjusted to the patient's level of knowledge and understanding, and the team should be particularly sensitive to her social, cultural, religious, ethnic, and economic origins. Education for health should cover nutrition, exercise, work, sexual activity, and the need to avoid tobacco, alcohol, and other drugs during pregnancy. Breast feeding should be discussed.

Regular exercise should be encouraged during pregnancy. Brisk walking is especially good. Activities such as swimming, jogging, and tennis may be continued by those accustomed to these types of activities; however, prolonged or strenuous aerobic exercise should not be undertaken.

Childbirth education classes provide an excellent opportunity for women to learn specific information relating to childbirth. Families should be encouraged to participate in childbirth education programs.

Education for childbirth may be provided in the physician's office, although more formal childbirth and parenthood classes may be offered by hospital or community agencies. Such classes should be planned and conducted by professionals. It is particularly important that physicians and obstetric nurses participate in these programs, because such participation fosters continuity of care and consistency of instruction. Those providing childbirth education should give expectant parents an opportunity to become familiar with the hospital's maternity and newborn units. This may be accomplished by a tour of the facilities or by audiovisual presentations.

Occupational Considerations

The patient's status in relation to her occupation should be reassessed throughout pregnancy. Based on the occupational history obtained during the initial evaluation, she should be given recommendations on minimizing potential hazards, including advice on whether she should continue working or make adjustments in her schedule.

When the potential hazards of the work environment are no greater than those encountered in normal daily life in the community, a woman with an uncomplicated pregnancy may continue to work without interruption until the onset of labor. Physical and emotional stress and environmental health hazards should be taken into consideration. Each case should be evaluated individually in determining degrees of disability of pregnancy that could interfere with a woman's ability to work.

Consideration should be given to the pregnant woman's health so she can modify her lifestyle and occupation as needed on a temporary basis. The physician may find it helpful to consult with occupational health care providers. Their experience and knowledge of the work responsibilities and environment can supply useful information. In addition, they can often help arrange job modifications that permit the patient to continue working. The physician should not seek such a consultation, however, without the patient's permission.

Psychosocial Services

Confronting psychological and social problems, such as fear of pregnancy, guilt associated with an unwanted pregnancy, financial concerns, and marital or other family conflicts, may be the most distressing part of a woman's pregnancy. A woman with negative feelings about her pregnancy needs additional support from the health care team, and she may need professional advice on the alternatives to completing the pregnancy and keeping the baby. Family members and their interactions with the pregnant woman should be considered in whatever recommendations are made.

The obstetrician should be alert to the stresses that may arise from the patient's psychological and social conflicts to ensure the early detection and effective management of emotional problems. The physician should be aware of individuals and community agencies to whom patients can be referred for additional counseling and assistance when necessary.

Adolescent Pregnancy

The physician should be prepared to assist the pregnant adolescent with conflicts that may arise, especially if the pregnancy is unplanned.

Family and social relationships may be seriously disturbed, and the adolescent, her family, and her friends may have strong feelings regarding the pregnancy. The physician can do much to ease tensions through counseling, education, and the use of community and social resources.

Once pregnancy has been confirmed, the physician should explore with the adolescent her feelings about the pregnancy and the options available to her. Late confirmation may complicate these considerations, however, and limit the options for management. The adolescent should take an active role in the decision-making process, and the physician should direct recommendations specifically toward her needs. Sensitive, perceptive, and in-depth discussions with the patient and those supporting her may be necessary.

POSTPARTUM EVALUATION

Postpartum review and examination should be accomplished 4–8 weeks after delivery. This interval should be modified according to the needs of the patient. The first postpartum review should include an interval history and physical examination to evaluate the patient's current status. This should include an assessment of weight and blood pressure, as well as breasts, abdomen, and external and internal genitalia. Laboratory data should be obtained as indicated.

The postpartum examination is an appropriate time for review of family planning; for immunizations, including rubella if not done immediately postpartum; and for discussion of any special problems. The patient should be encouraged to return for subsequent periodic examinations.

Based on the postpartum examination, the physician can determine if the woman is ready both physiologically and psychologically to resume working. Most women may return to work several weeks after an uncomplicated delivery. A period of 6 weeks is generally required for a woman's physiologic condition to return to normal, but the physician's recommendations on when the patient can resume full activity should be modified according to the patient's individual circumstances.

ADMINISTRATION

MEDICAL RECORDS

Each patient should have a medical record that includes both antepartum and in-hospital care data. A standard data base is desirable, and it is advisable that a common record be used within a community. The antepartum record should provide documentation of the history, physical examination, laboratory tests, and risk identification. Other pertinent data include an assessment of the course of pregnancy, identification of the patient's health needs, and plans for management.

The medical record is an important vehicle for communication among all members of the health care team. It should be legible, concise, cogent, and complete and should allow for easy assessment of the care provided to determine if the patient's health care needs have been identified, diagnosed, and effectively managed.

A copy or abstract of the current ambulatory care medical record should be available in the labor and delivery area of the hospital by the estimated 36th week of pregnancy, and arrangements should be made to obtain the record as soon as possible if admission prior to this time is necessary. Upon discharge from the hospital, the patient's ambulatory care record should be updated to include information on in-patient care pertinent to her subsequent management and the discharge summary if appropriate.

The record should be kept confidential and protected against fire, theft, and other damage for the duration of time prescribed by law or regulations, by good medical practice, or by state statute of limitations for personal injury.

QUALITY ASSURANCE

Professional personnel in the ambulatory care facilities should assess whether the health care provided has been effective and efficient. This may be done by including the care given in the ambulatory setting in the hospital patient care evaluation or by internal evaluations within the ambulatory setting. Health care evaluation should focus on the effectiveness of patient care and efficiency of resource use. It should include assessments of the completeness of the medical records, accuracy of diagnoses, appropriateness of the use of the laboratory and other services, and outcome of care. It should also include identification of potential problems in the care of patients, objective assessment of their cause, and designation of mechanisms to eliminate them. Efficient use of medical resources can be documented by evaluating use of personnel, finances, equipment, and facilities.

Obstetricians should practice ongoing review and comparison of their own experiences with standards of patient care and office practices suggested by the scientific literature, continuing medical education programs, or other obstetricians practicing in a similar circumstance.

PERSONNEL

The efficient operation of ambulatory care facilities requires adequate administrative and professional personnel to provide optimum care and safety, as well as to prevent undue delays in delivery of care. Obstetric care requires a team of professionals directed by a physician. In addition to an obstetrician, the team may include other physicians, certified nurse-midwives, nurse-practitioners, registered nurses and other nursing personnel, social workers, and nutritionists. Written policies describing the specific responsibilities of each member of the team are essential for larger facilities and desirable for all others, even the physician's office. The performance of each member of the health care team should be evaluated periodically.

It is advisable to hold regularly scheduled staff meetings to maintain effective communication and to provide periodic reviews of policies and procedures. There should be an ongoing program for in-service training of personnel appropriate for the facility providing care.

FACILITIES AND EQUIPMENT

The physical facilities and equipment described in the following sections are included to serve as guides for physicians' offices and outpatient clinics. Facilities and equipment may vary according to the type of practice and patient volume.

The reception area should have comfortable seating, patient education materials, and conveniently located rest rooms. There should be some provision for privacy in discussing confidential information, and for storing records with security and confidentiality.

A comfortable area should be provided for interviews and for counseling with the patient or her family. The physician's office may serve as a consultation room. Separate rooms, other than the physician's office, should be available for use by nurses, social workers, health educators, or other members of the health care team.

The following equipment should be available in the examining room area, but not necessarily in each room:

- Biopsy instruments
- Microscope
- Sphygmomanometer
- Stethoscope
- Fetoscope
- Ultrasonic fetal pulse detector

- Measuring tape
- Reflex hammer
- Ophthalmoscope
- Scale
- Supplies for obtaining
    Wet slide preparations and bacterial smears
    Specimens and cultures
    Cytologic studies

The exact number of examining rooms depends on the patient load; however, a minimum of two examination rooms is desirable. The following equipment should be available in each examining room:

- Screening to permit patient privacy
- Handwashing facilities
- Examination table with suitable disposable cover, and a stool
- Examination light
- Gynecologic examination equipment and supplies
- Work counter or table
- Small desk, table, or shelf for writing
- Storage cabinet

The utility room area should be equipped with the following items:

- Work counter
- Handwashing facilities
- Sink
- Closed cabinets for storage
- Locked medicine cabinets
- Refrigerator
- Facilities for sterilization unless central sterilization is available
- Waste receptacle

When local anesthesia is used, the following equipment should be available for possible emergency resuscitation:

- Positive pressure device and a source of oxygen
- Intravenous equipment and fluids
- Suction
- Laryngoscope and assorted airways

For larger practices or clinics, a conference and patient education room is desirable and may contain the following items:

- Comfortable chairs

- Conference table
- Educational materials and pamphlets
- Chalkboard
- Bulletin board
- Teaching models and equipment for demonstration
- Screen
- Slide projector
- Movie projector
- Videotape equipment

Specific plans and procedures outlining the following points should be established for the health and safety of patients and personnel:

- Methods for controlling electrical hazards and preventing explosion and fire
- Procedures for controlling and disposing of needles, syringes, glass, knife blades, and contaminated waste supplies
- Methods for storing, preparing, and administering drugs
- Plans for handling reasonably foreseeable emergencies, including methods for transferring a patient to a nearby hospital
- Plans for emergency patient evacuation and the proper use of safety, emergency, and fire-extinguishing equipment
- Plans for training of personnel in cardiopulmonary resuscitation
- Plans for adequately maintaining and cleaning facilities

3
Obstetrics: Hospital Care

The hospital setting, with either a traditional labor and delivery suite or a birth center, provides the safest environment for the mother and the baby during labor, delivery, and the postpartum period.

The scope of obstetric services offered by hospitals will vary with the patient volume and the level of care provided. Any facility providing obstetric care, however, should have the following minimum services available:

- Identification of high-risk mothers and fetuses
- Continuous electronic fetal monitoring
- Cesarean delivery capabilities within 30 minutes
- Blood and fresh frozen plasma for transfusion
- Anesthesia on a 24-hour basis
- Radiology and ultrasound examination
- Neonatal resuscitation
- Laboratory services on a 24-hour basis
- Consultation and transfer agreement
- Nursery
- Data collection and retrieval

Hospitals that serve as referral centers for high-risk obstetric patients will offer more and varied services than will hospitals that generally provide care only to low-risk patients.

Regardless of the patient volume or level of care provided, hospitals with obstetric patients should have facilities for the evaluation of antepartum complications requiring hospitalization, the care of patients during labor and delivery, and the postpartum care of patients and their babies. The inpatient obstetric service should be consolidated in a designated area, ideally an area that is physically separated from other patient care areas. The service should be staffed and equipped to handle obstetric and neonatal emergencies.

All hospitals with obstetric services should have access to a neonatal intensive care unit. Facilities without an intensive care nursery should establish procedures and methods for the transportation of sick neonates to a regional neonatal unit. When possible and practical, obstetric patients with complications likely to result in a sick or premature neonate should be transferred to a facility with a neonatal intensive care unit for delivery.

The laboratory facilities should have a 24-hour capability to provide blood group, Rh type and cross-matching, and basic emergency laboratory evaluations. Either ABO Rh-specific or O Rh-negative blood should be available at the facility at all times. Other laboratory procedures, such as serologic testing and determination of rubella titers, should be available.

ANTEPARTUM SERVICES

When the patient volume warrants, a high-risk antepartum care unit should be developed to provide facilities and nursing care for the mother and fetus at risk. When this is not feasible, it is desirable that an area in the postpartum unit be established for the care of sick or high-risk patients. Written policies should indicate where pregnant patients with obstetric, medical, or surgical complications should be assigned.

Facilities needed to monitor the status of the mother or the fetus will vary with the seriousness of the particular disease process, its known risk, and the care the hospital is prepared to provide. Services may include ultrasonography, electronic fetal heart rate monitoring, amniocentesis, and special laboratory tests to monitor maternal and fetal well-being.

Hospitals routinely serving low-risk obstetric patients may not find it economically feasible to provide ultrasonography, but this procedure should be available at a referral facility. Obstetric services caring for high-risk patients should be equipped to provide ultrasonography during labor and on a 24-hour basis. This diagnostic service should be under the direction of a physician who has a special interest in obstetric diagnoses and complications. Technical personnel should be trained in the obstetric application of ultrasound.

Equipment for electronic fetal heart rate monitoring, such as non-stress and stress testing of the fetoplacental unit, should be available for antenatal evaluation. Physicians using electronic fetal monitoring for antenatal surveillance must understand the indications, limitations, and interpretation of these tests.

Amniocentesis to establish fetal maturity or measure amniotic fluid optical density should be available. Small obstetric units may choose to refer patients when amniocentesis is indicated. Amniocentesis performed in early pregnancy for the purpose of genetic evaluation may require special handling of the specimen for accurate results. The genetics laboratory should be consulted for specific instructions.

ADMISSION POLICIES AND PROCEDURES

Obstetric patients with pregnancy induced hypertension, bleeding, premature rupture of the membranes, multiple gestation or other complications who require admission prior to the onset of labor should be admitted to the antepartum area. When the complication is serious and acute, the patient should be assigned to an area, such as the labor area, where she can receive more intensive observation and care.

Ideally, obstetric patients with a medical or suspected surgical condition complicating pregnancy should be assigned to the obstetric area. If a patient is critically ill, however, admission or transfer to an intensive care unit, in or away from the obstetric area, may be indicated. When the critically ill patient recovers sufficiently, she should be returned to the obstetric area, provided her care or the care of the other obstetric patients is not jeopardized.

Written policies and procedures should be established for the management of pregnant patients with known infectious illnesses.

INITIAL EVALUATION

The condition of every patient admitted to the antepartum unit should be evaluated by a physician. The evaluation should include a complete history of the present illness, past medical history, and family and social history. The extent of the physical examination to be performed and laboratory studies to be obtained depends on the condition of the patient and the reason for admission. A copy or abstract of the prenatal record should be available as soon as possible.

When a consultation is involved, the consulting physician is responsible for the pertinent history and those portions of the physical examination relevent to the consultation.

INTRAPARTUM SERVICES

Every obstetric service, regardless of size, should have written policies and procedures that indicate the areas of responsibility of both medical and nursing personnel for normal and emergency care. These policies and procedures should be reviewed yearly and made available to all department members. There also should be written policies for the care of pregnant patients when all antepartum and postpartum beds are occupied.

ADMISSION POLICIES AND PROCEDURES

Patients in labor, or those with premature rupture of membranes or with vaginal bleeding should be admitted directly to the labor and delivery suite. Occasionally, obstetric patients who are not in labor but require special intensive care may also be admitted to this area. A preadmission examining area should be available in the labor and delivery area for triage of all patients.

The admission of the patient in prodromal labor with no complications may be deferred to allow her to wait in a more casual, comfortable area. Under no circumstances should a patient be sent home without the knowledge of her physician.

The care of patients suspected of having a transmissible infection should be managed according to established hospital policy. Patients with urinary tract infections or low-grade postpartum fevers do not require isolation.

Nonobstetric Patients

The labor and delivery area may be used for nonobstetric patients during periods of low occupancy. Use of the delivery room for clean gynecologic cases is acceptable when staffing and equipment are adequate. Labor and delivery patients must take precedence over nonobstetric patients, however. The obstetric department, in conjunction with the hospital administration, should establish specific policies indicating which patients in addition to labor patients may be admitted to the labor and delivery suite. Procedures that may be performed in the delivery room include the following:

- Dilatation and curettage for noninfected spontaneous abortions
- Dilatation and curettage for induced abortions
- Dilatation and curettage of noninfected gynecologic patients
- Cerclage for cervical incompetence
- Sterilization
- In vitro fertilization-retrieval and implantation procedures

Evaluation and Preparation

Evaluation of the condition of every patient admitted to the labor and delivery area should consist of an updated history and an updated physical examination. This may be performed by a physician or a specially trained nurse. A copy of the ambulatory care prenatal record should be reviewed and filed in the patient's hospital record. Laboratory data should include blood group, Rh type, serologic tests for syphillis, rubella titer, and other laboratory data as indicated. A routine blood type and screen does not need to be repeated at the time of hospital admission for labor and delivery if it was performed during the antepartum period and did not indicate the presence of antibodies, if the report is on the hospital records, and if the patient does not have an increased risk for a blood transfusion.

The interval history should include time of onset of contractions, status of the membranes, and presence of any significant bleeding. Additional information should include time and content of the last oral intake, drug ingestion, known allergies, use of contact lenses or eyeglasses, and presence of dentures. Admitting personnel should note whether the patient attended childbirth education classes, her wishes regarding analgesia or anesthesia, and her plans for breast- or bottle-feeding.

The admitting physical examination should include the patient's blood pressure, pulse, and temperature. The fetal heart rate, as well as the frequency, duration, and quality of the uterine contractions, should be recorded. If there is suspected leakage of amniotic fluid or any unusual bleeding, the attending physician should be notified immediately—before a pelvic examination is performed. The degree of cervical dilatation, effacement, fetal presentation and position, and the station of the presenting part should be recorded. When there are no complications or contraindications, qualified nursing personnel may perform the initial pelvic examination. The physician responsible for the patient's care should be informed of her status, so that a decision can be made regarding further management.

Since there are no medical indications for routine perineal preparation and cleansing enemas, they should be performed at the discretion of the physician.

Childbirth is a unique family experience. The father of the baby, the family, or other support persons should have the opportunity to participate in the process within the realm of good obstetric care.

LABOR SURVEILLANCE

After the patient in labor has been admitted and her status has been evaluated, ongoing intrapartum surveillance is necessary. The degree and method of observation vary according to predetermined risk factors. A qualified member of the obstetric team should be assigned responsibility for observing the patient, following her progress in labor, and recording all pertinent information, such as vital signs and fetal heart rate, on the labor record. The physician responsible for the patient's care should be kept apprised of her progress and notified immediately of any abnormalities.

Any new significant symptoms or signs, such as excessive vaginal bleeding or meconium staining, should be evaluated by the physician. In most cases, assessment of the quality and frequency of uterine contractions, determination of the fetal heart rate, and performance of a pelvic examination should be adequate to detect evidence of any abnormality and to assess the progress of labor. If a complication arises, it should be recorded and the patient should be informed of its nature and implications.

Maternal temperature should be recorded at least every 4 hours, and more often if indicated. Maternal blood pressure should be measured and recorded every hour and immediately prior to delivery. Hypertensive patients require more frequent blood pressure determinations. The amount of fluid intake and output should be recorded.

In the first stage of labor, the fetal heart rate should be ascultated and recorded at least every 30 minutes. This evaluation is best carried out immediately following a uterine contraction. In the second stage of labor the fetal heart rate should be evaluated and recorded at least every 15 minutes. When the patient is prepared for delivery, the fetal heart rate should be checked at least every 10 minutes. The fetal heart rate should also be evaluated immediately after rupture of the membranes.

It is desirable for hospitals with a labor and delivery service to have the capability of continuous electronic fetal monitoring. Continuous electronic monitoring of fetal heart rate and uterine activity during labor is recommended for patients with significant risk factors. Electronic fetal monitoring is highly sensitive but has low specificity; therefore, on the basis of fetal heart rate patterns alone, definitive cause and effect relationships between patterns and long-term outcome cannot be determined. When electronic fetal heart rate monitoring is used, the physician and obstetric personnel are responsible for its interpretation. If monitoring suggests fetal distress that does not respond to conservative measures, the infant should be delivered expeditiously.

The monitor tracings are a part of the medical record, and, although the tracings need not be stored with the record, they should be readily retrievable. The tracings should include the patient's name and hospital number and date and time of admission and delivery. Relevant data, such as examinations, changes in position of the patient, and medications and corresponding times, should be recorded on the tracings.

Although its exact role is controversial, fetal capillary pH can be a useful adjuvant to intrapartum fetal assessment. The procedure is a reasonable option in the appropriate setting.

The use of intravenous fluids and medications for analgesia and anesthesia depends on the judgment of the attending physician. The routine use of medications is not recommended.

MEDICAL INDUCTION OR AUGMENTATION OF LABOR

Induction or augmentation of labor with oxytocin may be initiated only after a responsible physician has evaluated the patient, determined that induction or augmentation is beneficial to the mother or fetus, recorded the indication, and established a prospective plan of management. Only a physician who has privileges to perform cesarean deliveries should initiate these procedures. A physician or qualified nurse should examine the patient vaginally immediately prior to the oxytocin infusion.

A written protocol for the preparation and administration of the oxytocin solution should be established by the obstetric department in each institution. Oxytocin should be administered only intravenously, with a device that permits precise control of the flow rate. While oxytocin is being administered, an electronic fetal monitor should be used for continuous recording of fetal heart rate and uterine contractions.

Personnel who are familiar with the effects of oxytocin and able to identify both maternal and fetal complications should be in attendance while oxytocin is being administered. A qualified physician should be readily accessible to manage any complications that may arise during infusion.

DELIVERY

When delivery is imminent, the patient should not be left unattended, nor should any attempt be made to delay the birth of the infant by physical restraint or anesthesia. At least one member of the nursing staff should be in the delivery room throughout the delivery. During delivery, the maternal blood pressure and pulse should be evaluated at least every 10 minutes and recorded. If electronic fetal monitoring is not being used or has been discontinued, the fetal heart rate should be evaluated by auscultation and recorded at least every 10 minutes. The maternal blood pressure and pulse should be evaluated immediately after delivery and at least every 15 minutes during the first hour and thereafter until the patient's condition is stable.

When continuous electronic fetal heart rate monitoring has been used during labor, the following guidelines are recommended for fetal evaluation in the delivery room until vaginal delivery occurs:

- If previous tracings have been normal, continued surveillance may be conducted with auscultation. The findings should be recorded at least every 10 minutes. If delivery does not occur in the anticipated time, continuous electronic fetal monitoring should be reestablished.
- If the tracings have been abnormal, electronic fetal monitoring should be reestablished unless delivery is imminent or is being expedited, (i.e., in response to fetal distress, when taking time to reestablish electronic fetal monitoring could cause unnecessary delay).

If internal monitoring is being used in patients who undergo cesarean delivery, the scalp electrode should be left attached to the fetus and the monitoring equipment until the abdominal preparation is complete. If external monitoring is used, it should be continued until the abdominal preparation is begun.

Postpartum orders should be noted by the physician on the patient's chart. Routine postpartum orders may be used, but they should be printed or written on the chart, reviewed and modified as necessary for the particular patient, and signed by the physician before the patient's transfer to the postpartum unit.

When a birthing room is used, the same standards of care should apply as in a traditional setting.

ANESTHESIA

In any hospital with an obstetric service, a person qualified to administer anesthesia should be readily available to administer an appropriate anesthetic and to maintain support of vital functions in any emergency. In larger facilities caring for high-risk patients, 24-hour, in-house anesthesia coverage is strongly recommended.

The anesthesiologist or anesthetist should be informed in advance if a complication with the delivery is anticipated. Anesthesia information discussed during her prenatal care should be reviewed with the patient, including information regarding the advantages, disadvantages, and risks associated with the various forms of anesthesia.

An obstetrician trained in anesthesia administration may provide the anesthesia if such privileges have been granted by the obstetric and anesthesia departments. It is preferable, however, for an anesthesiologist or anesthetist to provide this care so that the obstetrician may devote undivided attention to the delivery. All obstetricians should be trained in the use of infiltration anesthesia.

When regional anesthesia is administered by the obstetrician, the patient should be monitored by a qualified member of the health care team. Maternal blood pressure should be taken every 5 minutes for the first 15 to 20 minutes or until the patient is stable and thereafter periodically as indicated during the anesthesia administration. All vital signs and the patient's status should be recorded on a standard anesthesia record. Intravenous fluids should be started before the induction of any general or regional anesthesia.

FATHERS IN THE DELIVERY ROOM

Fathers and support persons may be permitted in the delivery room with the consent of the obstetrician and the patient. A dress code that conforms to that of the professional personnel in the delivery room should be followed. Fathers or support persons should be adequately informed of the normal events and procedures in the labor and delivery area. They should understand that their major function is to provide psychologic and physical assistance to the mother during the labor and delivery process. Whether the support person may be present at cesarean birth depends on the judgment of the obstetric staff, the individual obstetrician, the anesthesiologist, and the policies of the hospital. A written policy is recommended.

IMMEDIATE CARE OF NEWBORN

The person who delivers the baby is responsible for the immediate postdelivery care of the newborn until another qualified person assumes this duty. Routine care of the healthy newborn is often delegated to appropriately trained nurses.

Recognition and immediate resuscitation of the distressed infant requires an organized plan and immediate availability of equipment and qualified personnel. The directors of obstetrics, anesthesia, pediatrics, and nursing should jointly plan the provision of resuscitation services, and the plan should have the approval of the medical staff. They should also develop a list of maternal and fetal conditions that require the presence in the delivery room of someone specifically qualified in newborn resuscitation. A physician must be designated to assume primary responsibility for the establishment of standards of care, review of practices, maintenance of appropriate drugs, and training of personnel. Planning must include specific identification and immediate in-house availability of qualified personnel on a 24-hour basis.

The newborn should be examined for any abnormalities, and the Apgar scores should be determined, evaluated, and recorded. Care of the newborn's eyes and the umbilical cord and identification of the newborn should be carried out according to written hospital procedures and local statutes.

If the parents desire circumcision of the newborn, it is recommended that this be performed subsequent to the infant's stabilization period following birth.

POSTPARTUM SERVICES

The time mother and baby spend in the hospital after delivery is a very important part of the obstetric experience. Policies and procedures should be established for identifying and managing any postpartum complications that may arise.

INITIAL RECOVERY CARE

Following delivery, the patient should be constantly attended and closely observed for postpartum complications. Vital signs, including pulse, respiration, and blood pressure, should be recorded at least every 15 minutes during the first hour and thereafter until the patient's condition is stable. Fluid intake and output should be recorded. The uterine fundus should be frequently examined to determine if it is well contracted and to check for excessive bleeding.

The patient's physician should be notified of any significant changes in her vital signs, excessive vaginal bleeding, or any other unusual findings. The patient should remain in the recovery area for at least 1 hour or until she has recovered from anesthesia. Patients recovering from major conduction or general anesthesia should be discharged at the discretion of the attending physician or anesthesiologist in charge of the recovery area. Similar care should be provided for the patient who uses the birthing room. Nursing personnel assigned to observe postpartum patients should be qualified to recognize postpartum emergencies and problems as they occur and should have no other obligations. Generally, the father or other support person may be allowed to remain with the mother in the recovery area. Parents may be given an opportunity to interact with the infant unless maternal or neonatal complications prevent it. When the baby is allowed to remain with the mother, the infant should be closely observed for any abnormal signs. Once the patient's vital signs have been stabilized, she may be transferred to her room in the postpartum area.

Patients who deliver outside the hospital should be examined in the labor and delivery suite prior to being admitted to the postpartum recovery area.

POSTPARTUM CARE

After the patient has been transferred to her room, her vital signs, the status of the fundus, and bleeding should be reassessed and recorded. The assessment should be repeated at regular intervals for the next several hours. The unsensitized Rho(D) negative patient who has delivered an Rh positive infant should receive Rh immune globulin as early as possible in the postpartum period, preferably within 72 hours, even if she has received prophylatic Rh immune globulin prenatally at 28 weeks of gestation. If a patient has been determined to be susceptible to rubella, she should receive rubella vaccine prior to discharge.

A specific family-centered plan for patient education is an important element of postpartum care. The mother should receive instructions in caring for herself and her baby. Group or individual sessions may be held regularly for patients during the postpartum period to teach and discuss self-care; breast examination; infant care, including breast and bottle-feeding, bathing, growth, and development; parent-infant relationships; family planning; and exercise. Specific postpartum policies and procedures should be established through cooperative efforts of the medical and nursing staffs.

New mothers with infectious illness may be housed in single rooms on the postpartum floor or in another area of the hospital. If the disease is likely to be transmitted to the baby, the mother and the newborn should be separated until the disease is no longer communicable. Patients whose temperature elevation is known to be due to a nontransmissible infection or a low-grade postpartum infection may be kept on the obstetric unit, and there is no need to separate them from their newborns. Patients suspected of having a transmissible infection should be managed according to established hospital policy.

VISITING

The father and other support persons may be with the patient as much as desired during the labor, delivery, recovery, and postpartum periods, subject to the constraints of hospital facilities, policies, and acceptable standards of care.

It may be desirable for children to visit their mother during the postpartum period, especially children under 6 years of age who may experience anxiety when separated from their mother. Some hospitals have designated sibling visiting areas, while others permit visiting in the rooms of postpartum patients. The father or another adult should accompany the siblings and assume responsibility for their care and conduct.

Allowing the siblings to see the newborn in the hospital can help to prepare them for the new family member. Direct contact with the newborn is acceptable if the siblings have no infectious disease and infection control procedures are followed. Exposure of the newborn to children other than the siblings should be avoided.

Other family members and friends may be allowed to visit the patient and see the newborn in accordance with hospital facilities, policies, and acceptable standards of care.

DISCHARGE PLANNING

The purpose of the postpartum stay is to keep the patient under observation long enough to identify maternal and infant complications, to provide professional assistance during the time when the mother is most apt to be uncomfortable, and to educate the parents about child care enough so that they may return home with reasonable competence and confidence. Each patient should be adequately instructed regarding normal postpartum events, care of breasts and perineum, care of the urinary bladder, amounts of activity allowed, diet, exercise, emotional response, family planning, resumption of coitus, and signs of common complications. She should also be instructed regarding baby care and subsequent newborn medical examinations.

Arrangements for postpartum follow-up evaluation should be made at the time of discharge, and the patient should be given information on what to do if a complication or an emergency arises. With shortened postpartum stays, it is particularly important to emphasize the roles of the obstetrician, pediatrician, and other members of the health team in the continuing care of both the patient and her infant.

EARLY DISCHARGE

Although most women whose deliveries were uncomplicated are discharged with their infants in 48 to 72 hours, earlier discharge may be desired. Plans for early discharge should be discussed in the antepartum period. The family and physician should discuss the criteria to be met, and a plan should be outlined with the concurrence of the pediatrician. In case of an early discharge, especially within 24 hours of delivery, the following conditions should be met:

- The mother should have had an uncomplicated vaginal term delivery following a normal antepartum course and should have been observed after delivery for a sufficient time to ensure that her condition is stable. Pertinent laboratory data, including hemoglobin or hematocrit, ABO determination, and Rh determination should have been obtained. Rh immune globulin should have been given if indicated.
- The newborn should be normal and stable; sucking and swallowing abilities should be normal. Routine medical evaluation of the neonate's status at 2–3 days of age should have been arranged.
- Family members or other support individuals should be available to the mother for the first few days following discharge.
- The mother should be aware of possible complications involving either herself or the infant and should have been instructed to notify the appropriate practitioner as necessary.

USE OF OBSTETRIC BEDS FOR NONOBSTETRIC PATIENTS

There should be a written policy regarding the use of obstetric beds for nonobstetric patients. Such admissions should not compromise the care of obstetric patients. The use of obstetric beds is permissible if the following guidelines are observed:

- An adequate number of obstetric beds must always be available to accommodate peak volumes.
- The physician responsible for the obstetric service should have the final authority in determining which nonobstetric patients are admitted.
- Only patients with noninfectious conditions should be admitted. No patient who is febrile at the time of admission or who

may be reasonably suspected of infection should be admitted to a bed in the obstetric area.

- Visiting hours and rules for nonobstetric patients should not interfere with the normal function of the obstetric unit.
- Nonobstetric patients should be admitted only if the obstetric nursing staff can adequately provide care for them without detracting from the care of obstetric patients.
- Admission of nonobstetric patients should conform to local and state regulations.

ADMINISTRATION

MEDICAL RECORDS

Every patient should have a medical record that includes a copy of the prenatal record or an abstract of the current record of ambulatory health care as well as in-hospital data. The medical record should also indicate transfer to and from another facility because of risk factors necessitating additional services at another level of care.

Like the ambulatory care record, the hospital record serves as a vehicle for communication among all members of the health care team. It should be legible, concise, cogent, and comprehensive. Furthermore, it should permit an easy assessment of care provided and should reflect the patient's current status. The hospital record should contain the following information:

- Patient identification data
- Prenatal record
- Interval history and physical examinations
- Provisional diagnosis to include preoperative diagnosis if applicable
- Diagnostic and therapeutic orders
- Physicians' and nurses' notes
- Laboratory data
- Informed consent
- Labor and delivery record
- Operative report
- Anesthesia report
- Medications record
- Discharge instructions
- Discharge summary

The check-off type of discharge summary may be used for normal cases. All significant complications; operative deliveries, including all cesarean deliveries; and fetal conditions, such as serious morbidity or stillbirth, should have an individually written or dictated discharge summary. A copy of the summary should become part of the patient's ambulatory care record.

Maternal and newborn records should be compared and studied in tandem to evaluate care from ambulatory prenatal care through labor, delivery, and newborn outcome.

QUALITY ASSURANCE

Every hospital should have a quality assurance program to assess whether management of health care and use of resources have been effective and efficient. Evaluation of patient care should include assessments of the completeness of medical records, the accuracy of diagnoses, appropriateness of use of laboratory and other services, and outcome of care. It should also include the identification of important or potential problems in the care of patients, the objective assessment of the causes of these problems, and the designation of mechanisms or actions to eliminate them insofar as is possible. An evaluation of the use of personnel, finances, equipment, facilities, and length of patient stay determines the efficiency of medical resources used.

The staff of each department of obstetrics should continually evaluate the patient care it provides, using reliable and valid written criteria. The evaluation team should consist of individuals knowledgeable in methods of quality assurance review as well as in the topic being reviewed. Process or outcome audit may be used as one form of assessment of the quality of care rendered.

Each hospital should have a utilization review program to enable proper allocation of its resources without compromising the quality of patient care. There should be a written plan of review, and members of the obstetric patient care team should be involved in the performance of all resource reviews.

Each maternal death and selected perinatal deaths should be reviewed in detail, including an evaluation of postmortem findings. Maternal and neonatal morbidity and complications should be reviewed periodically.

The quality assurance program should be evaluated periodically to ascertain whether it fosters effective patient care, satisfactory professional performance, and cost efficiency.

PERSONNEL

The efficient operation of an obstetric facility requires adequate staffing with both administrative and professional personnel. The medical head of the obstetric service, in conjunction with the nursing manager of the obstetric services is responsible for organizing and supervising the antepartum, labor and delivery, and postpartum units. Staffing levels that provide for optimum patient care and safety are determined by the number of patients, patient profile, type of procedures, and the design of the facility. A mechanism should be established for calling in additional staff during peak patient census.

Obstetric care requires a team of professionals directed by a physician. In addition to an obstetrician, this team may include an anesthesiologist, a pediatrician, family physician, certified nurse-midwife, nurse-practitioner, registered nurse, other nursing personnel, nutritionist, and social worker. Written descriptions outlining the responsibilities of these personnel should be prepared and reviewed periodically. Each member's performance should be evaluated periodically.

There should be ongoing programs of in-service training for personnel with special emphasis on policies, current medical practice, and practice technique. Team personnel should also hold regular patient care planning meetings.

FACILITIES AND EQUIPMENT

The physical facilities of an obstetric service should provide a safe and comfortable environment in which women can give birth and care for their infants. Ideally, the inpatient obstetric service should be consolidated in an area that is physically separate from the rest of the hospital, such as on a floor, in a wing, or in a separate building. Physical arrangement, however, is determined by the number of patients and available space. Every effort should be made to make facilities flexible and to meet local needs.

The size and type of service will determine whether antepartum, intrapartum, and postpartum units are separate or combined. Some hospitals provide rooms in which these services are combined, enabling labor, delivery, and recovery to take place in one area without the need to transfer patients.

The following facilities should be available to both antepartum and postpartum units and, in appropriate circumstances, may be shared:

- Nurses' station
- Physician and nurse charting area

- Conference Room
- Nurses' lounge
- Patients' lounge
- Patient education area
- Examination and treatment room(s)
- Secure area for storage of medications
- X-ray view boxes
- Instrument cleanup area
- Area and equipment for bedpan cleansing
- Sitz bath facilities
- Kitchen and pantry
- Workroom and storage
- Sibling visiting area
- Sterilization equipment (if central sterilization equipment is not available)

Equipment and supplies should include the following items:

- Stretchers with side rails
- Equipment and facilities for pelvic examinations
- Sphygmomanometers and stethoscopes
- Fetoscopes
- Fetal monitoring equipment
- Supplies for examining urine for sugar and protein
- Needles and syringes
- Solutions and equipment for administering parenteral fluids
- Equipment for obtaining blood specimens
- Emergency drugs
- Suction apparatus, either wall outlet or portable equipment
- Urinary catheterization equipment
- Cardiopulmonary resuscitation cart to include
  Needles
  Syringes
  Emergency drugs
  Laryngoscope
  Airways
  Equipment for delivering positive pressure oxygen
  Adult cardiac monitor
  Suction apparatus, if not otherwise provided
  Defibrillator
- Ice machine

Additional facilities and equipment for inpatient and outpatient testing of the mother and fetus vary with the level of care the hospital is prepared to give. Hospitals with a special intensive care section should be able to accomplish the following procedures:

- Ultrasonography
- Fetal monitoring, e.g., nonstress and stress testing
- Maternal monitoring, e.g., continuous cardiac and venous pressure
- Amniocentesis
- Cardiopulmonary resuscitation

Patients who have significant medical or obstetric complications requiring intensive observation and care should be placed in a room especially equipped with monitors, supportive electromechanical devices, and cardiopulmonary resuscitation equipment. If the room is located in the labor and delivery area, it should meet the physical standards of any other intensive care room in the hospital, and the standard of care provided should be equivalent to that of the intensive care unit.

Antepartum

The antepartum unit should provide comfort, privacy, and protection against infection, as well as an atmosphere conducive to rest.

Each patient unit should include the following items:

- Bed with adjustable side rails
- Adequate lighting
- Bedside stand
- Space for clothes and personal belongings
- Signal or intercommunication device
- Bathing, toilet, and handwashing facilities
- Screening of beds in multiple-bed rooms

Intrapartum

There should be a separate area for patient examination and short-term observation. There should also be a comfortable waiting area with nearby rest rooms adjacent to the delivery suite.

Labor Rooms. In order to provide patient privacy, there should be a labor room for each patient. Each room should have immediately adjacent toilet and handwashing facilities, which may be shared with an adjoining room, and an emergency call system. The room should have a minimum of 140 square feet of usable space for support persons, personnel, and equipment. Doorways should be large enough to accommodate the labor bed. The labor room may also function as a delivery or birthing room, recovery room, or an intensive care unit for high-risk patients.

The following equipment is recommended for each labor room:

- Labor or birthing bed
- One or more comfortable chairs
- Adjustable lighting that is adequate for examinations and pleasant for the patient
- Emergency signal and an intercommunications system
- Adequate ventilation and temperature control
- Auxiliary electric system
- Sphygmomanometer and stethoscope
- Mechanical infusion equipment
- Fetal monitoring equipment
- Oxygen and suction outlets
- Writing surface for charting
- Storage facilities

Delivery Rooms. To ensure easy access, the delivery rooms should be located close to the labor rooms, but they should be away from the entrance to the labor and delivery suite. There should be no traffic through the delivery rooms. The number of delivery rooms needed depends on the average number of deliveries per day, although every delivery unit should have at least two delivery rooms. Small obstetric services may consider equipping a labor room for alternate use as a delivery room.

The traditional delivery room is similar in design to an operating room. The size of the room should accommodate the equipment and personnel needed for either vaginal delivery or cesarean delivery. Each room should be well lighted and environmentally controlled, and there should be an auxiliary electrical system. At least one delivery room should be equipped with an operating table and instruments for cesarean deliveries. It is highly desirable that cesarean deliveries be performed in the delivery unit; postpartum sterilization may also be performed there.

Each delivery room should be maintained as a separate unit with equipment and supplies necessary for normal delivery and management of complications:

- A delivery table that allows variation in position for delivery
- Instrument table and solution basin stand
- Adequate lighting for vaginal delivery or cesarean delivery
- Instruments and equipment for vaginal delivery, repair of lacerations, cesarean delivery, postpartum sterilization, and cesarean hysterectomy
- Solutions and equipment for administering intravenous fluids

- Equipment for inhalation and regional anesthesia
- Heated, temperature-controlled infant examination and re-suscitation unit
- Equipment for examination and identification of the infant
- Resuscitation equipment, including laryngoscope, endo-tracheal tubes, and breathing bags for term and preterm infants
- Oxygen and suction outlets for mother and infant
- An emergency call system
- Mirrors for patients to observe the birth
- Wall clock

Scrub sinks with arm, knee, or foot controls should be strategically placed so that the physician who is scrubbing can observe the patient.

Clean gynecologic operations may be performed in the delivery rooms if patients are adequately screened to eliminate infectious cases and if personnel are sufficient in number to keep the quality of obstetric care from being compromised. The medical head of the department of obstetrics and gynecology should be responsible for final patient selection. It is recommended that these selected clean gynecologic operations be performed in a designated, properly equipped delivery room and that these patients be observed in a recovery room.

Labor/Delivery/Recovery Rooms. Combined units should be designed to provide services available in separate units while at the same time enhancing the woman's comfort and permitting the family's interaction with their newborn. Each combined room should be equipped with the following items:

- Labor/delivery bed
- Bedside table
- Closet
- One or more comfortable chairs
- Emergency signal and intercommunication system
- Oxygen and suction outlets
- Adequate ventilation and temperature control
- Adjustable lighting system
- Sink
- Mirrors for the patient to observe the birth
- Wall clock
- Fetal monitoring equipment

Birthing Rooms. To accommodate those low-risk patients who want to deliver their babies in a more homelike setting but to have hospital services immediately available should they be needed, a birthing room may be used. The area should be a combined waiting-labor-delivery area where family members or other support persons may remain with the patient as much as possible throughout the childbirth process. It should be located in or close to the intrapartum area.

Furnishings should be bright, attractive, and homelike. The room should otherwise contain the same equipment and supplies as do other labor and delivery rooms, preferably concealed in wall cabinets or behind drapes. Equipment for electronic fetal monitoring and anesthesia should be accessible from the intrapartum area. The room should contain a unit for maintaining the baby's temperature or for warming the infant and administering oxygen.

If a problem arises for which treatment cannot be administered appropriately without moving the patient, steps should be taken for immediate transfer of the patient to a traditional unit. Facilities for cesarean delivery should be readily available.

The birthing room should be under the supervision of the medical head of the department of obstetrics and gynecology, and personnel who work in the unit should be subject to all the rules and regulations of the department.

On-Call Rooms and Lounges. Separate lounges with locker rooms and rest rooms should be provided for physicians and nurses. Individual sleeping facilities for physicians on call should be located near the delivery area. Where applicable, a sleeping area for the house staff and students should be available.

Postpartum

Each patient unit should be equipped with the following items:

- Bed
- Adequate lighting
- Bedside stand
- Space for clothes and personal belongings
- Signal or intercommunication device
- Bathing, toilet, and hand-washing facilities
- An emergency call signal
- Screening of beds in a multiple-bed room

When rooming-in is permitted, each room should have hand-washing facilities, a bassinet unit, and supplies necessary for the care of the newborn.

4
Gynecology: Ambulatory Care

MEDICAL SERVICES

The gynecologist providing ambulatory gynecologic medical services is frequently called on to balance the roles of principal care physician and specialist. For most women, the gynecologist is the only physician providing continuity of care. When principal care is provided, a comprehensive examination should be performed at various intervals throughout a woman's lifetime. The frequency of such an examination depends on the woman's lifestyle, the risk of disease at various times of her life, and environmental factors.

The gynecologist should provide a continuum of gynecologic health care. The physician should take into consideration the needs of the woman for information and education about health maintenance, developing and changing sexuality, family planning, genetic risk of reproduction, and specific medical and surgical conditions related to gynecology. The physician should encourage breast self-examination and should make each patient aware of common health risks to which she may be vulnerable at various times of her life. Patient education may include explanations of anatomy and physiology, as well as instructional material and demonstrations such as methods of breast self-examination. The important role of the individual in her health care should be stressed.

As a part of a woman's overall health care, the gynecologist should recognize the patient's sexual, psychologic, and social needs. The physician should identify areas of difficulty and, when necessary, should involve community services available for patient and family support.

INITIAL GYNECOLOGIC EVALUATION

A woman should have a gynecologic examination by at least the age of 18 years. Sexually active women should have periodic examinations regardless of their age.

Following are the recommended basic components of the initial gynecologic evaluation:

History

- Purpose of the visit
- Present illness

- Menstrual and reproductive history
- Medical, surgical, emotional, social, family, and sexual history
- Medications
- Allergies
- Family planning
- Systems review

Physical examination

- Height, weight, nutritional status, blood pressure
- Head and neck, including thyroid
- Heart
- Lungs
- Breasts
- Abdomen
- Pelvis (external and internal genitalia)
- Rectum
- Extremities
- Lymph nodes

Laboratory

- Urine screen
- Hemoglobin or hematocrit
- Cervical cytology
- Rubella titer (reproductive age group)

Other laboratory studies should be performed if indicated by physical findings, history, and risk factors.

PERIODIC GYNECOLOGIC EVALUATION

All aspects of the data base established at the initial evaluation should be updated periodically. Current practice is to perform the appraisal on asymptomatic women annually, although this interval may be modified as indicated by a woman's health risk and the therapeutic regimens used. Following are the recommended basic components of the periodic gynecologic evaluation:

History

- Purpose of the visit
- Menstrual history
- Interval history, including systems review
- Emotional history

Physical examination

- Weight, nutritional state, blood pressure
- Thyroid
- Breasts
- Abdomen
- Pelvis (external and internal genitalia)
- Rectum
- Other areas as indicated by the interval history

Laboratory

- Urine screen
- Cervical cytology

Additional laboratory tests should be performed, as indicated, based on the history, physical examination, and risk factors.

CANCER SCREENING

Periodic updating of the woman's health history and an examination of the thyroid, breasts, abdomen, pelvis, and rectum are important in cancer screening. The frequency of this screening should be determined by the risk status of the woman. Beginning at 18 years of age, younger if they are sexually active, most women should undergo cervical cytology evaluation annually. It is particularly important that high-risk women, i.e., those who have had early sexual intercourse and those who have had several sexual partners or multiple marriages, be screened annually. It may be desirable for women over 40 years of age to be screened for colon and rectal cancer by testing for occult blood. Any abnormal findings should be further evaluated.

BREAST DISEASE

Examination of the breasts is an essential part of the initial and periodic physical examination. The obstetrician-gynecologist should take a major role in detecting breast disease and in teaching women the importance and methods of breast self-examination. The patient should be questioned about her knowledge of breast self-examination and whether she has detected signs or symptoms of breast disease. The physician should be alert to changes influenced by a woman's age, menstrual cycle, parity, pregnancy, and body habits.

The physician should investigate any abnormality, such as nipple discharge, cyst formation, or solid mass. Obstetrician-gynecologists may manage cyst aspiration and surgical removal of solid tumors in accordance with their training and experience.

Although inspection and palpation remain important diagnostic approaches for the detection and diagnosis of breast lesions, mammography has significantly increased the physician's ability to deal with breast disease. Mammography should be considered for women with breasts that are difficult to examine and for those with persistent nipple discharge, dominant breast mass, a personal history of breast malignancy or a family history of breast malignancy in a mother or sister, or first pregnancy after age 30. Mammography should also be considered when a lump is felt by the patient but cannot be confirmed by the physician and when the breast has been altered by augmentation procedures. A baseline mammogram is recommended for women between the ages of 35 and 50 years.

FAMILY PLANNING

The physician should make available to patients information on reproductive physiology, methods of fertility control, and sterilization. Family planning services should be offered within a context of comprehensive counseling, including human sexuality and the prevention of sexually transmitted infections. Where appropriate, family planning services should be integrated into regular gynecologic care to allow continued observation.

Another aspect of family planning is preconceptional counseling. This can help determine the advisability and timing of pregnancy, assess and possibly stabilize risks, and reinforce good health and lifestyle habits that are conducive to pregnancy. This type of counseling before conception can help promote the well-being of the fetus during the first several weeks of gestation when a woman may not be aware she is pregnant.

A general medical and gynecologic history, with physical examination and appropriate laboratory studies, should be used to evaluate the relative or absolute contraindications to specific family planning methods for a particular patient. It is important to establish the level of the patient's knowledge about reproductive physiology and about her specific needs. She should be made aware of the availability, effectiveness, and relative risks of different methods. Conception control is the responsibility of both partners; both male and female methods should be considered.

The sexually active adolescent girl deserves special attention because of the high incidence of unintended pregnancy in this population. The gynecologist should attempt to ensure that she has access to the most suitable methods of contraception.

In the event of an unwanted pregnancy, the physician should counsel the patient about her options of continuing the pregnancy to term and keeping the infant, continuing the pregnancy to term and offering the infant for legal adoption, or aborting the pregnancy. When possible, and with the patient's approval, the physician should offer this counseling to her partner and to her parents if she is a dependent adolescent, before these difficult decisions are made. If the patient elects abortion, she should be counseled for future reference that abortion is not recommended as a primary method of family planning. When pregnancy termination is recommended by the physician for medical or psychiatric indications, consultation may be appropriate.

STERILIZATION

When a woman elects to undergo surgical sterilization, she should be fully aware of the implications of the operation. As a part of her informed consent, the woman should express her understanding that the procedure is intended to be permanent, that there can be no guarantee of the effectiveness of the procedure, and that restoration of fertility by a subsequent operation is uncertain.

If sterilization is requested by the patient and her physician agrees to perform the surgery, consultation is not necessary. If medical or psychiatric problems complicate the decision for sterilization, however, the opinion of a knowledgeable consultant may be desirable.

ENDOCRINE DYSFUNCTION AND INFERTILITY

Infertility and reproduction endocrine disorders in women, such as dysfunctional uterine bleeding, amenorrhea, hirsutism, and galacorrhea, are frequently encountered in gynecologic practice. Modern gynecologic training and continuing education provide the gynecologist with an adequate basis for investigation and management of most of these problems.

Infertility management requires the evaluation of both partners. Although the woman will be the gynecologist's primary focus, he or she may undertake the initial evaluation of the male as well. Comprehensive evaluation and treatment of the male should be done by a physician with training or experience in male infertility.

General medical, nutritional, urologic, gynecologic, and endocrine disorders may all play a role in infertility. In the female, consideration should be given to cervical, uterine, ovarian, and tubal factors. Management of the infertile couple demands sensitivity, not only to the couple's organic problems, but also to their emotions. Factors that involve both partners, particularly those related to coitus, should be evaluated. The results of the evaluation and the treatment plan should be discussed with both partners. Referral may be indicated in complex situations requiring skills, knowledge and techniques of ovulation induction, sperm antibody assessment, tubal repair, in vitro fertilization and embryo transfer.

PEDIATRIC AND ADOLESCENT GYNECOLOGY

It is appropriate for a gynecologist to care for a female infant, child, or adolescent with a gynecologic problem. A data base should encompass not only a gynecologic history but also a general medical history. The complete physical evaluation should include an examination of the external genitalia and a digital rectal examination. The nature of the patient's problem determines whether a vaginal and cervical examination should be included. Adequate time should be allowed to deal with the patient's anxieties and needs. In the assessment of a young patient, it is important to include an evaluation of nutrition, pubertal development, and sociosexual adaptation. The gynecologist should offer the sexually active adolescent information regarding human reproduction and sexuality, sexually transmitted disease, and fertility control.

SEXUAL ASSAULT

The obstetrician-gynecologist can play a vital role in the care of the patient who has been sexually assaulted. Sensitive evaluation and care should be provided.

The physician's primary responsibility is to treat the patient, to prevent disease, and to consider the possibility of pregnancy. Since every instance of alleged sexual assault can lead to legal action the physician should note both positive and negative findings, including signs of injury in the medical record.

Prior to examination, separate consent forms should be obtained for the examination and for taking photographs and gathering evidence. A systematic approach to the examination is essential to locate any injuries that should be noted and photographed. Proper evidence, including history, physical findings, laboratory study results, specimens, clothing, and photographs, should be gathered, and custody of evidence should be documented.

Since the emotional trauma of sexual assault may be as great as, if not greater than, the physical injury, early emotional support and counseling by qualified, sensitive persons are imperative. Immediate and long-term follow-up support and counseling are essential to help the victim and her family cope with resultant emotional and social problems. If the patient is a minor, State laws may require the physician to report the incident to government authorities.

It is important for the health care team to recognize its role and responsibility in helping the victim's family and other significant persons to cope with the crisis. The family, or others emotionally close to the victim, can affect how well the patient copes with short- and long-term effects of the assault.

SEXUAL COUNSELING

Within the context of sexual counseling, it is important to recognize the broader aspects of sexuality, including interpersonal relationships, sexual adjustments, and lifestyles. A sexual history is an important part of a comprehensive health inventory. The gynecologist should provide an opportunity for the patient to discuss her concerns about sexuality. A patient checklist may be useful in initiating this communication. If a patient has a problem beyond the scope of the physician's expertise, or if the physician is ill at ease in this role, referral should be made to an appropriate consultant.

GENETIC COUNSELING

The gynecologist should be alert to any indication of genetic disorders or conditions that might lead to birth defects. Screening for the detection of potential genetic disorders begins with a careful history of family, drug, and environmental factors. Inquiries should be made about the outcome of previous pregnancies, mental retardation, or other known or suspected inherited or metabolic disease. Whenever possible, disorders should be diagnosed prior to pregnancy. When a genetic disorder is suspected, the gynecologist should discuss with the patient the ways in which the genetic disorder may affect her health, her reproductive capabilities, or the development of her offspring. When counseling a couple with a suspected genetic abnormality, the gynecologist should provide the information necessary for the patient to decide, based on the potential social, emotional, and economic consequences, whether to proceed with further investigation. The gynecologist may wish to refer patients with potential genetic disorders to qualified genetic counseling and evaluation centers.

SURGICAL SERVICES

Certain surgical procedures may be performed on an ambulatory basis to conserve time and expense for the patient and to use hospital facilities efficiently. A physician's office, an outpatient clinic, or a free-standing or hospital-based ambulatory surgical facility may be used. Procedures should be limited to those that can be performed safely within the constraints of staff expertise and physical facilities. If the patient has a major medical disorder, appropriate consultation should be obtained before proceeding with a surgical procedure in an ambulatory facility.

Informed consent should be obtained before any surgical procedure is performed. Upon discharge, the patient should be given adequate postoperative instructions, preferably written, and arrangements should be made for routine and emergency follow-up care. The importance of a follow-up evaluation should be stressed during both the preoperative and postoperative interviews.

Removed tissue should be submitted to a pathologist for examination. The patient should be informed of the operative findings, including the results of the tissue examination. After an elective termination of pregnancy, the attending physician should record a description of the gross products. Unless definite embryonic or fetal parts can be identified, the products of elective interruptions of pregnancy should be submitted to a pathologist for gross and microscopic examination.

PHYSICIAN'S OFFICE AND OUTPATIENT CLINIC

Only surgical procedures that can be performed either without anesthesia or with only local anesthesia may be performed in the physician's office or in an outpatient clinic. When local anesthesia is used in these settings, equipment and qualified personnel should be available for emergency resuscitation.

Procedures commonly performed in a physician's office or in an outpatient clinic include, but are not limited to, the following:

- Abortion, uncomplicated, up to 14 weeks from last menstrual period
- Aspiration of a breast cyst
- Biopsy, aspiration, or washing of the endometrium
- Cervical polypectomy
- Cervical, vaginal, and vulvar biopsies
- Colposcopy

- Cryosurgery, fulguration, or vaporization of the cervix or vulva
- Culdocentesis
- Cystometric studies
- Cystoscopy
- Dilatation and curettage
- Hysterosalpingography
- Hysteroscopy
- Incision and drainage of vulvar or perineal abscesses
- Evacuation of incomplete abortions, spontaneous and uncomplicated
- Insertion of intrauterine contraceptive device
- Proctosigmoidoscopy
- Removal of skin lesions
- Tubal insufflation
- Urodynamic studies
- Uterine sounding

FREE-STANDING AND HOSPITAL-BASED FACILITIES

Ambulatory surgical facilities that are free-standing or hospital-based should maintain the same surgical, anesthetic, and personnel standards that hospitals do. Surgical procedures may be performed in these facilities under general or regional block anesthesia when the postoperative recovery is expected to permit discharge on the same day.

Procedures commonly performed in a free-standing or hospital-based ambulatory surgical facility include, but are not limited to

- Breast biopsy
- Colpotomy
- Examination under anesthesia
- Extensive biopsies or extensive fulgurations of vulvar lesions
- Laparoscopy, including diagnostic procedures, tubal sterilization, or other surgical procedures if laparotomy is not anticipated
- Marsupialization of a Bartholin duct abscess or cyst
- Minilaparotomy for sterilization
- Simple perineoplasty
- Cervical conization

Those procedures performed in the physician's office or the outpatient clinic also may be performed in these facilities. There should be a written policy providing for prompt emergency treatment or hospitalization of patients in the event of an unanticipated complication.

A qualified anesthesiologist, another qualified physician, or a certified nurse-anesthetist under the supervision of an anesthesiologist, may administer general epidural or spinal anesthesia in an ambulatory surgical unit. When any form of anesthesia is used, trained personnel and proper equipment for cardiopulmonary resuscitation should be available. A physician, preferably the anesthesiologist, should be present in the ambulatory surgical facility until all patients have been discharged. This physician should oversee the postanesthetic recovery area and should share with the surgeon responsibility for discharging patients or transferring them to the back-up hospital.

Only a patient at low risk should be considered for ambulatory surgery. A preoperative history and physical examination should be completed no more than 2 weeks before the surgical procedure is to be performed. Preexisting or concurrent illness, medications, and adverse drug reactions that may have an effect on the operative procedure or anesthesia should be identified. Laboratory data should include hemoglobin or hematocrit, urine screen, and, in selected patients, other studies such as a chest x-ray, electrocardiogram, and determination of electrolyte levels. The patient should be given preoperative instructions, especially regarding the restriction of food and fluids, and advised that noncompliance can result in cancellation of the procedure.

On the day of surgery, a preanesthetic evaluation, including an interval history, medical record review, and heart and lung examination should be performed by a physician, and the findings should be noted in the record.

A recovery area is necessary. During the recovery period, a member of the health care team should observe the patient continuously. This person should maintain a complete record of the patient's general condition, including vital signs, blood loss, and occurrence of complications. The patient should remain in the area until recovery is sufficient to permit safe discharge in the company of a responsible adult.

Upon discharge, the patient should be given instructions about medications, her follow-up care, the signs and symptoms of common complications, and how to obtain emergency care and advice.

ABORTION

Ambulatory care facilities for abortion services should meet the same standards of care as for other surgical procedures. Physicians performing abortions in their offices should provide for prompt emergency treatment or hospitalization in the event of complication. Clinics and free-standing ambulatory care facilities should have written agreements with nearby hospitals for the transfer of patients requiring treatment for emergency complications in abortion procedures.

Generally, abortions in the physician's office or outpatient clinic should be limited to those performed within 14 weeks from the first day of the last menstrual period. In a hospital-based or free-standing surgical facility, abortions should be limited generally to those performed within 18 weeks from the last menstrual period. Prior to an abortion, the woman should be counseled on the options for management of an unwanted pregnancy. She should be allowed sufficient time for reflection prior to making an informed decision. If counseling has been provided elsewhere, the physician who is to perform the abortion should verify that the counseling has taken place.

In addition to the history, physical examination, and indicated laboratory procedures, an Rh factor and antibody screen should be performed. Every unsensitized Rho(D) negative woman who has an abortion should receive Rh immune globulin. Before the patient's release from the facility, aspirated tissue should be examined to ensure that villi or fetal parts are present. If villi or fetal parts are not identified with certainty, the tissue specimen should be sent for further pathologic examination and the patient alerted to the possibility of an ectopic pregnancy.

The patient should receive instruction in the use of family planning methods, and counseled that abortion is not recommended as a primary method of contraception.

ADMINISTRATION OF PHYSICIAN'S OFFICE AND OUTPATIENT CLINIC

MEDICAL RECORDS

Physicians' offices and outpatient clinics should maintain accurate medical records for each patient. The record should be legible, concise, cogent, and complete. In addition, the record should allow easy assessment of the care provided to determine if the patient's health needs have been effectively managed. Because medical practice frequently involves several physicians and other professionals and because the record serves as a vehicle for communication among all members of the health care team, it should be readily accessible.

All medical information should be confidential and the record secure. All records should be retained for the period of time prescribed by law and by good medical practice.

At the initial visit, a comprehensive data base and plan of therapy should be established and updated during each visit. Correspondence, operative notes, and laboratory data should be reviewed and filed chronologically in the patient's medical record. Any pertinent data regarding changes in health status or inpatient care should be recorded; this may take the form of a diagnostic summary.

QUALITY ASSURANCE

Personnel in each outpatient clinic and physician's office should assess the effectiveness and efficiency of health care management. In the outpatient clinic, evaluation of patient care should include assessments of the completeness of medical records, the accuracy of diagnoses, appropriate use of laboratory and other services, and outcome of care. It should include the identification of potential problems in the care of patients, the objective assessment of the cause of problems and designation of mechanisms to eliminate them. Efficient use of medical resources can be documented by evaluating use of personnel, finances, equipment, and facilities.

Gynecologists should periodically review their office practices, comparing it with standards of patient care and office practices suggested by the scientific literature and continuing medical education programs.

PERSONNEL

Administrative and professional personnel requirements in physicians' offices and outpatient clinics depend on the patient load, pattern of practice, and type of facility. The members of the health care team should participate in the specific areas of care according to their training and within written definitions of their responsibilities. Policies and responsibilities should be reviewed and revised periodically. Regular meetings of personnel should be encouraged, and there should be an ongoing program for in-service training.

FACILITIES AND EQUIPMENT

The physical facilities and equipment required depend on the type of practice and patient volume, but certain items should be reasonably available for the care of patients within the office or clinic setting. For example, the reception area should have comfortable seating, patient education materials, and conveniently located rest room facilities. Sufficient space should be provided to ensure that medical and financial records are handled and stored with security and confidentiality.

A comfortable and private area should be provided for interviews and for counseling with the patient or her family. The physician's office may serve as a consultation room. Separate rooms, other than the physician's office, should be available for use by nurses, social workers, health educators, and other members of the health care team. Equipment for each consultation room should include at least a desk or table with two chairs.

The following equipment should be accessible to, although not necessarily in, each examining room:

- Biopsy instruments
- Instruments for vaginal and rectal examinations
- Microscope
- Sphygmomanometer
- Stethoscope
- Reflex hammer
- Ophthalmoscope
- Scale
- Supplies for obtaining
    Specimens and cultures
    Wet slide preparation and bacterial smears
    Cytologic studies
- Equipment necessary for diagnostic studies and operative procedures performed in the facility

When local anesthesia is used, the following equipment should be available for emergency resuscitation:

- Positive pressure device and a source of oxygen
- Intravenous equipment and fluids
- Suction
- Laryngoscope with assorted airways

The exact number of examining rooms required depends on the patient load and type of practice; however, even a solo physician's office should have at least two examination rooms. The following equipment should be available in each examining room:

- Screening to permit patient privacy
- Handwashing facilities and paper towels
- Examination table with suitable disposable cover and a stool
- Examination light

- Gynecologic examination equipment and supplies
- Work counter or table
- Small desk, table, or shelf for writing
- Storage cabinet

The utility room area should contain the following facilities:

- Work counter
- Handwashing facilities and paper towels
- Sink
- Cabinets for storage
- Locked medicine cabinets
- Refrigerator
- Facilities for sterilization unless central sterilization is available
- Waste receptacle

For larger practices or clinics, a conference and patient eduction room may contain the following items:

- Comfortable chairs
- Conference table
- Educational materials and pamphlets
- Chalkboard
- Bulletin board
- Models and demonstrating equipment
- Screen
- Slide projector
- Movie projector
- Video equipment

Specific plans and procedures for the health and safety of patients and personnel should include the following information:

- Methods for controlling electrical hazards and preventing explosion and fire
- Procedures for controlling and disposing of needles, syringes, glass, knife blades, and contaminated waste supplies
- Methods for storing, preparing, and administering drugs, when applicable
- Plans for handling reasonably foreseeable emergencies, including methods for transferring a patient to a nearby hospital
- Plans for emergency patient evacuation and the proper use of safety, emergency, and fire equipment

- Plans for training of personnel in cardiopulmonary resuscitation
- Plans for adequately maintaining and cleaning the facilities

ADMINISTRATION OF FREE-STANDING AND HOSPITAL-BASED AMBULATORY SURGICAL FACILITIES

MEDICAL RECORDS

All ambulatory facilities should maintain an accurate and efficient record system. The records used should conform to a standard record used in the community or back-up hospital. All medical information should be secure, confidential, and readily accessible. The record should be legible, concise, cogent, and complete. Furthermore, the record should facilitate assessment of the care provided to determine if the patient's health needs have been identified, diagnosed, and managed effectively. The patient's record should include details in regard to any anesthetic used, the procedure performed, any difficulties encountered, and the patient's subsequent condition. Because modern medical practice frequently involves several physicians and professionals, the record should serve as a vehicle for communication among all members of the health care team.

This record should contain sufficient information not only to justify the preoperative diagnosis and the operative procedure, but also to document the postoperative course. The record should contain the following information:

- Patient identification data
- History and physical examination findings
- Provisional diagnosis
- Diagnostic and therapeutic orders
- Surgeon's and nurses' notes
- Laboratory results
- Operative consent
- Operative report
- Anesthesia report
- Tissue report
- Medications record
- Discharge note and instructions

The record should be completed promptly and signed by the attending physician. A discharge note should be written or dictated. The ambulatory care facility should keep registries of admissions and discharges, operations, and controlled substances. Records should be kept confidential and should be protected against fire, theft, and other damage for the duration of time prescribed by law and by good medical practice.

QUALITY ASSURANCE

The effectiveness of patient care and the use of the ambulatory surgical facility should be continually evaluated. A team of professionals qualified to assess all aspects of patient care, including completeness of medical records, accuracy of diagnoses, and outcome of care, should be responsible for evaluating patient care. The evaluation should include identification of potential problems in the care of patients, objective assessment of their cause, and designation of mechanisms to eliminate them. Particular care should be taken to identify ambulatory treatments that might have been undertaken more appropriately on an inpatient basis.

PERSONNEL

The efficient operation of an ambulatory surgical facility requires that administrative and professional personnel be assigned on the basis of the number of patients, patient profiles, types of procedures performed and facility design. Written policies describing the specific responsibilities of each member of the team are desirable and should be reviewed and revised periodically. There should be an ongoing program for in-service training of personnel.

The governing body of the ambulatory surgical facility has the final authority and responsibility for the appointment of the medical staff. Privileges should be granted only to those who are properly trained, have been licensed, and have demonstrated competence. These privileges should not exceed those granted to the same individual in at least one accredited hospital within the geographic area.

FACILITIES AND EQUIPMENT

The general physical design for a free-standing or hospital-based ambulatory surgical facility depends on the number and types of surgical procedures to be performed. The facility should provide a comfortable, safe environment with minimal architectural barriers. Traffic flow should be convenient and efficient. A multilevel facility should have elevators that can accommodate stretchers.

The facility should include space adequate for the following functions:

- Reception and waiting
- Administrative activities, such as patient admission, record storage, and business affairs
- Patient dressing and lockers
- Preoperative evaluation, including physical examination, laboratory testing, and preparation for anesthesia
- Performance of surgical procedures
- Preparation and sterilization of instruments
- Storage of equipment, drugs, and fluids
- Postanesthetic recovery
- Staff activities
- Janitorial and utility support

The instruments, equipment, and supplies used in the ambulatory surgical facility should be equivalent to those used for similar procedures in an accredited hospital and should provide for the following:

- Control of sources and transmission of infection
- Infection surveillance
- Functional oxygen and suction
- Resuscitation and defibrillation
- Emergency lighting
- Sterilization
- Emergency intercommunication

Specific plans and procedures should be established for the health and safety of patients and personnel. Such plans and procedures should include the following information:

- Methods of control against the hazards of electrical or mechanical failure, explosion, and fire
- Comprehensive emergency plans, including but not limited to patient evacuation and the proper use of safety, emergency, and fire extinguishing equipment
- Equipment and personnel for handling reasonably foreseeable medical emergencies arising from services rendered
- Provision for transferring unanticipated emergency cases to a nearby backup hospital
- Training of personnel in cardiopulmonary resuscitation

- Control and disposition of needles, syringes, glass, knife blades, and contaminated material
- Proper storage, preparation, and administration of drugs
- Facilities that are accessible, barrier-free, and safe for all, including the handicapped
- Adequately maintained and clean facilities

5
Gynecology:
Hospital Care

SERVICES

Inpatient gynecologic care consists of integrated medical and surgical services for the diagnosis and treatment of conditions that involve the female reproductive tract and require the patient to be hospitalized. The scope of services provided varies according to the training and interest of the attending gynecologists, the size and accessibility of the facility, and the availability of laboratory facilities and special technology and equipment. High-quality care is more easily attained on a specialty service. When hospital size permits, the gynecologic inpatient service should be consolidated in one designated area. In smaller hospitals where the number of patients may not justify establishing a separate area, gynecologic patients may be treated in either a medical or surgical area. Noninfected gynecologic patients may be treated in the obstetric area when hospital policy permits and when it does not interfere with the operation of the obstetric unit. Nursing personnel caring for gynecologic patients should be familiar with special aspects of gynecologic conditions and equipment needed to care for these patients.

MEDICAL GYNECOLOGY

Women may require hospitalization for treatment of pelvic infection, evaluation of endocrine disorders, and chemotherapy and irradiation for gynecologic malignancies. In each of these areas, the gynecologist is by training and experience usually the most qualified to manage the patient's treatment. When the problems are more complex or beyond the skill and knowledge of the attending gynecologist, however, they should seek appropriate consultation.

When radioactive and other dangerous materials are part of the therapeutic regimen, special provision should be made for the protection of the patient, other patients, and attending personnel. The hospital should have written policies and protocols for the use of these therapeutic modalities, and personnel working with these materials should have special training and skills in their use, including knowledge of necessary protective measures and, when required, proper disposal techniques.

GYNECOLOGIC SURGERY

Although limited primarily to the female reproductive system, gynecologic surgical services cannot be rigidly defined. Variations in local practice are determined largely by the special skills of physicians available in the community. Each hospital, with the approval of the department of obstetrics and gynecology, should establish its own regulations in accordance with the training and experience of the individual members of the gynecologic staff.

Gynecologists who perform major abdominal surgery should be able to manage injury or disease involving adjacent structures, such as bowel, bladder, and ureter. Those without such surgical skill should request consultation with other specialists in the management of these problems. Likewise, other surgical specialists who encounter gynecologic complications should seek gynecologic consultation with problems that lie outside of their usual surgical experience. Gynecologists may perform diagnostic and therapeutic urologic procedures in the lower urinary tract to the extent of their training and experience. Patients with gynecologic malignancies should be treated by the gynecologist. If the therapy is complex, consultation with or referral to a gynecologic oncologist or a gynecologic oncology team may be warranted.

Tissue removed surgically should be submitted to a pathologist for examination. The patient should be informed of the results. An exception to the routine pathologic examination of tissue may occur in elective terminations of pregnancy in which embryonic or fetal parts can be identified. In such instances, the physician should record a description of the gross products. If definite embryonic or fetal parts cannot be identified, the products of elective interruptions of pregnancy should be submitted to a pathologist for gross and microscopic examination, and the patient alerted to the possibility of an ectopic pregnancy.

Competent assistants should be available for all major gynecologic operations. Nonphysician personnel may serve as first assistants if the obstetric-gynecologic staff has accepted the concept of nonphysician assistants and if that individual has completed an appropriate training program and has been approved by the hospital administration.

ADMISSION POLICIES AND PROCEDURES

All gynecologic patients admitted to the hospital should have a complete history including a menstrual history, and a physical examination recorded on the chart. The results of the most recent cervical cytology evaluation should also be noted in the patient's hospital record. The extent of diagnostic laboratory testing, such as a complete blood count, electrocardiogram, chest x-ray, electrolyte determination, and blood type and screen, should be individualized for the patient's problem and her age. Basic laboratory evaluation prior to a surgical procedure should include a hemoglobin or hematocrit and a urinalysis.

Patients scheduled for surgical procedures who are at risk of appreciable blood loss should have a blood group and Rh type determination and screening for antibodies. The presence of antibodies should be reported by the blood bank, since it requires specific cross match. When the surgeon anticipates blood loss requiring replacement, blood (or components) should be cross matched and available for the patient's use.

An Rh factor determination should be made of every patient scheduled for pregnancy termination, and Rh immune globulin should be administered to every unsensitized Rho(D) negative woman following the termination.

PREGNANCY EVALUATION

Since many diagnostic and therapeutic modalities may pose a direct or indirect risk to an embryo, hospitals should establish specific procedures, applicable to all services, for identifying unsuspected pregnancies in hospitalized women of reproductive age. A menstrual history and physical examination can be helpful in this determination. If there is any reason to suspect pregnancy, a pregnancy evaluation should be done.

HEALTH EDUCATION

Patient education is an integral part of disease prevention and management. All members of the health care team should help the woman and her family understand her illness and treatment plan. The patient may have concerns about her disease and how its treatment may affect her reproductive function and her sexuality. Explanations should be given to allay these anxieties.

The patient should be given any necessary instructions for self-care, including special diets, self-administration of medications, good health habits, breast self-examination, and personal hygiene.

DISCHARGE PLANNING

Early in the patient's hospitalization, discharge planning should be initiated. The health care team should formulate an individualized plan that takes into account the needs and desires of the patient and her family, as well as the community resources available. On discharge, the patient should be given instructions, preferably written, about medications, follow-up care, activity restrictions, exercise, resumption of coitus, the symptoms and signs of common complications, and how to obtain emergency care and advice. The roles of other physicians and members of the team concerned with the patient's health care should be delineated.

ADMINISTRATION

MEDICAL RECORDS

The medical record is a primary requisite for good patient care. Since it serves as a vehicle for communication among all members of the health care team, it should be legible, logical, concise, cogent, and comprehensive. The record should permit an easy assessment of whether the patient's health care needs have been identified, correctly diagnosed, and effectively managed. A problem list should be developed from the information obtained from the history, physical examination, and laboratory data. A problem-oriented approach is recommended for recording medical information.

Each record should contain the following applicable information:

- Patient identification data
- History and physical examination findings
- Provisional diagnoses
- Diagnostic and therapeutic orders
- Physicians' and nurses' notes
- Laboratory data
- Informed consent
- Operative report
- Anesthesia report
- Tissue report
- Discharge instructions
- Diagnostic summary
- Discharge summary (except for short-stay admissions)

The history should include the following information:

- The reason for admission
- Menstrual history
- Obstetric history

- Gynecologic history
- Method of fertility control
- Past medical and surgical history
- Current medications
- Allergies
- Social history
- Family history
- Review of systems

The discharge summary should include a brief review of the following information:

- Reasons for admission
- Significant findings
- Treatment rendered
- Procedures performed
- Complications
- Condition of the patient at the time of discharge
- Medications to be continued
- Follow-up care recommended
- The final diagnoses, including any histopathologic diagnoses

A copy of the summary should be filed in the patient's ambulatory care record and sent to the physician who is to provide her follow-up care.

QUALITY ASSURANCE

Each hospital should have a quality assurance program to assess the effectiveness and efficiency of health care management and resource use. Evaluation of patient care should include an assessment of the completeness of medical records, accuracy of diagnoses, appropriateness of use of laboratory and other services, and outcome of care. It should also include the identification of potential problems in the care of patients, the objective assessment of the cause of these problems and the designation of mechanisms or actions to eliminate them as far as possible. An evaluation of personnel, assignments, finances, equipment, facilities, and length of patient stay determines the efficiency of use of medical resources.

Each department of gynecology should continually evaluate the patient care it provides, using reliable and valid written criteria. The review team should consist of members of the department of obstetrics and gynecology who are knowledgeable in methods of quality assurance review as well as in the topics being reviewed. A process or outcome audit may be used as one form of assessment of the quality of care rendered.

Each hospital should have a utilization review program to enable proper allocation of its resources without compromising the quality of patient care. There should be a written plan of review, and members of the gynecologic staff should be involved in the performance of all resource reviews.

PERSONNEL

A team of professionals, directed by a physician, may be organized to provide more effective care to patients with gynecologic problems. Members of the team should participate in the specific areas of care according to their training and within the hospital's written definition of their responsibilities. Written position descriptions outlining responsibilities should be prepared and reviewed regularly. The performance of each staff member, including each physician, should be evaluated periodically. Credentials of each physician should be reviewed according to policy.

The medical head of the gynecologic service, in conjunction with the nursing manager of the gynecologic service, is responsible for organizing and supervising the care of patients admitted for operative and nonoperative care. The assignment of personnel should be based on the number of patients, patient profile, types of procedures performed, and facility design.

The written patient care policies of the gynecologic service should be reviewed and revised periodically. There should be an ongoing program of inservice education for personnel, with special emphasis on service policies, current medical practice, and practice technique.

FACILITIES AND EQUIPMENT

Each patient unit should be equipped with the following items:

- Bed with adjustable side rails
- Bedside stand
- Space for clothes and personal belongings
- Screening of beds in multiple-bed rooms
- Signal or intercommunication device
- Bath and toilet facilities with emergency call system
- Comfortable chair

Whenever possible, each room should have its own toilet and washing facilities.

Wherever female patients are admitted, specific provisions should be made for pelvic examinations to be done privately and without delay. The examination room should be readily accessible and equipped with the following items:

- Proper screening to permit patient privacy
- Handwashing facilities and paper towels
- Examination table with suitable disposable cover and a stool
- Examination light
- Gynecologic examination equipment and supplies
- Work counter or table
- Small desk, table, or shelf for writing
- Storage cabinet

Equipment and supplies available to the gynecologic unit should include the following items:

- Equipment for performing examinations, biopsies, wound dressings, and paracentesis
- Speculums of various sizes, including those for pediatric patients
- Stretcher with rails
- Sphygmomanometer and stethoscope
- Materials for cytologic smears and bacterial cultures
- Supplies for obtaining urine specimen
- Equipment for obtaining blood specimens
- Intravenous infusion equipment
- Emergency drugs
- Suction, either by wall outlet or by portable equipment
- Cardiopulmonary resuscitation with
    Needles
    Syringes
    Emergency drugs
    Laryngoscope
    Airways
    Equipment for delivering positive pressure oxygen
    Cardiac monitor
    Defibrillator

6
Special Considerations

DATA COLLECTION

A significant portion of any quality assurance program is devoted to the study of outcome of obstetric-gynecologic procedures and practices. Standardized definitions are essential to accurate communications among health care personnel. Standardization is also pertinent to the development of a data base that allows comparison of effectiveness of services among institutions, of individual institutions to regional and national norms, and of changes within an institution over a period of time. The data base derived by a uniform approach to the study of outcome is a valuable component of the continuing education of health care personnel and provides a focal point for instituting change with the objective of subsequent improvement in the effectiveness of health care services.

Information provided by institutions in a uniform manner allows for better health planning at state and national levels. Because of delays in reporting information, collating data and completing the feedback process, however, the centralization of information has inherent weaknesses in its usefulness to institutions in detecting deficiencies in the delivery of obstetric-gynecologic services. A planned, systematic, periodic review of performance within an institution, using a standardized information approach, provides an excellent mechanism for the evaluation of programs and services.

The use of standardized terminology, definitions, and statistic-gathering procedures is the key to clear, precise communication at all levels of health care.

To facilitate institutional review as part of an overall quality assessment program, availability of data concerning the following outcome criteria will be useful.

Obstetrics
  Live Births
  Fetal Deaths
    Early Fetal Deaths
    Late Fetal Deaths
  Maternal Deaths
  Cesarean Deliveries
    Primary Cesarean Deliveries

Maternal Morbidity
Neonatal Deaths
    Early Neonatal Death
    Late Neonatal Death
Gynecology
    Surgical Complications (See Appendix for Criteria.)

INFORMED CONSENT

It is the physician's responsibility to inform the patient of the nature of the surgical or medical procedure being recommended. In most cases, the explanation should include the necessity of the treatment, the management alternatives, the reasonably foreseeable risks and hazards involved, the chances of recovery, and the likelihood of desired outcome. Adequate opportunity should be provided to encourage and answer questions, including those regarding nonmedical issues such as cost. It is suggested that a physician make a notation in the patient's record indicating the information communicated.

PATIENTS' RIGHTS AND RESPONSIBILITIES

Recognition of the rights of patients is an important aspect of health care. Patients are entitled to the following rights:

- Impartial access to high-quality care
- Respect, dignity, and privacy
- Assurance of confidentiality of their disclosures and their records
- Knowledge of the identity and professional status of individuals providing their health care

Patients should be advised of their diagnosis, treatment, and prognosis, and given an opportunity for informed participation in their health care. Patients have the right to request consultation or to refuse treatment. In addition, they have the right to have an appropriate representative exercise these rights when they are unable to do so for themselves.

Patients have responsibilities as well. A patient is responsible for providing accurate and complete health information and for indicating whether she understands the contemplated plan of management and the kind of compliance expected of her. The woman must take responsibility for her actions if she refuses treatment or does not comply with the plan of management. The physician has the right to discharge from his or her care a patient who declines or fails to cooperate in the therapy offered, provided that appropriate notice is given and there is an adequate opportunity for her care to be obtained from another source.

RADIATION PRECAUTIONS

DIAGNOSTIC X-RAY EXAMINATION

Possible pregnancy should be a special consideration when obtaining abdominal diagnostic x-rays in any female of reproductive age. A history, physical examination, and laboratory studies when appropriate should be utilized to rule out the possibility of pregnancy before such x-ray examinations are obtained. Even when all reasonable attempts to discover pregnancy are made, women with undetected pregnancies will undergo diagnostic x-ray examinations. To date there are no data implicating usual diagnostic x-ray examinations as definitely harmful to the ovum or developing fetus. Such x-ray exposure should not, therefore, be used as a reason for therapeutic abortion in the absence of other indications.

THERAPEUTIC RADIATION

Only physicians who demonstrate the necessary education or experience in the use of ionizing radiation should be allowed to perform radiation therapy. All physicians and other professionals dealing with therapeutic radiation sources should have privileges from the governing body of the facility. Cooperation and consultation between the gynecologist and radiotherapist are essential in order to achieve optimal patient management.

The hospital should have comprehensive written policies, procedures, and safety rules to protect the patient, visitors, and hospital personnel. Written procedures should not only guide personnel in the safe use, removal, and storage of radiation sources, but should also provide for the periodic monitoring and recording of the radiation exposure of involved hospital personnel. Radiation safety policies should conform to the recommendations of recognized radiation protection agencies. The radiotherapist and the radiation safety committee should provide ongoing in-service education programs.

Documented, informed consent is an integral part of all forms of therapeutic radiation. A signed pathology report identifying the diagnosis of the tumor should be in the patient's record before any form of radiation therapy is instituted. A complete radiation therapy summary should be filed in the patient's chart, as well as a progress note completed by the responsible physician indicating the radiation source, duration of exposure, or time of application, and time of removal, and the total dose calculated to standard points of reference.

CONSULTATION

A consultant is a physician asked by the attending physician to provide advice on the diagnosis and management of a medical problem. The consultant may be a member of any department of the medical staff and should be recognized for knowledge and skills in the specialty area for which the consultation has been requested.

Requesting and providing consultation is a formal process that should be accomplished according to certain guidelines. The attending physician should submit to the consultant a written request that includes the reason for the consultation and any other pertinent information. The consultant should review the medical record, obtain any necessary additional history, examine the patient, and note findings and recommendations in the patient's record. The consultant should discuss all recommendations with the attending physician, who should convey the information to the patient. The consultant should not discuss the findings and treatment directly with the patient without the permission of the attending physician. Subsequent management should be the attending physician's responsibility.

Informal opinions do not fulfill the requirements of consultation. While such opinions may serve a valuable educational function, they should be discouraged for the purpose of individual patient management. When an emergency requires immediate definitive action, a verbal consultation may be provided. If this is necessary, the written opinion of the consultant should be promptly placed on the record.

Physicians and patients alike are encouraged to seek additional medical advice when there is doubt about the diagnosis or a course of treatment. However, the competent, concerned physician, caring for an informed patient, is best prepared to evaluate the appropriateness of surgery. The "mandated second opinion" fails to recognize that, when there is disagreement, the "second opinion" may not be better or in the best interest of the patient.

When the complexity of an illness, complication, or procedure exceeds the category of privileges of an attending physician, consultation should be required. It may be necessary to transfer the care of the patient to an appropriate physician. Local situations may make it advisable to designate specific conditions, complications, or procedures for which consultations are required.

Transfer of Responsibility

It is important to distinguish between consultation and transfer of responsibility for patient care. In consultation, a physician is asked to evaluate a patient's problem and to make recommendations concerning the diagnosis and management. The attending physician is expected to continue medical supervision. If the attending physician does not have the training or experience to provide indicated medical treatment, transfer of the patient to the care of a qualified physician is indicated.

Responsibility for initiating the transfer of patient care is the attending physician's. The transfer should be understood clearly by the patient, her family, hospital personnel, and the physician who is to assume responsibility. This information should be documented in the patient's hospital record.

Joint Responsibility

At times, by mutual agreement, the consultant may assume the continuing responsibility for a designated portion of a patient's care while the attending physician otherwise retains the general management of care, e.g., the division of responsibility between an obstetrician and a cardiologist in the care of an obstetric patient with heart disease. Each physician's responsibilities should be clearly understood not only by the physicians, but also by the patient, her family, and the other members of the health care team.

REGIONAL CONSULTATION AND REFERRAL SYSTEM

When local facilities are unable to provide for specialized management of patients with complicated or high-risk obstetric or gynecologic conditions, the physician should seek consultation through a regional consultation and referral system. After consultation has been obtained, the physician, the patient, and the patient's family should decide whether she should be treated locally or transferred to a regional center for specialized evaluation or management of her care. When a patient is referred to a regional center, the medical staff at the center should ensure that the referring physician continues to be involved in and apprised of the patient's progress. The transferred patient should be returned to her own physician's care as soon as is feasible.

OBSTETRICS

The obstetric services offered by smaller hospitals often depend on economic factors, geography, climate, and the availability of transportation.

The obstetrician should manage high-risk obstetric patients locally when local facilities and staff are adequate to ensure optimal outcome for mother and infant.

Adequate care of high-risk obstetric patients is dependent on the continuous availability of a coordinated team of physicians, support personnel, laboratory services, and equipment to provide specialized support and intervention. Such a team is most effective if it is frequently involved in the care of high-risk patients. When it seems likely that the neonate will require intensive or specialized care not locally available, the obstetrician should consider transferring the mother to allow delivery in a hospital with a neonatal intensive care unit. If this is the case, the referring physician should be kept apprised of the patient's status and provided copies of her medical record. Neonatal transport capabilities should always be readily available for instances in which antepartum transfer is impractical or when newborn illness is unanticipated.

GYNECOLOGY

The gynecologist should have access to consultation at regional centers where patients can be referred for unusual gynecologic conditions. These conditions, which usually fall into the areas of gynecologic oncology or reproductive endocrinology, may require specialized diagnostic, surgical, or therapeutic expertise that can be attained only through advanced training and long experience.

When it is anticipated that a disease process will require skill and resources beyond those locally available, the physician should refer the patient for consultation and possible transfer. The patient's care should be returned to the referring physician when consultation or special therapy has been completed.

PROFESSIONAL EDUCATION

Medical education is a continuous and necessary activity of obstetric and gynecologic departments. It may include continuing medical education, and undergraduate and graduate education.

CONTINUING MEDICAL EDUCATION

The hospital's department of obstetrics and gynecology should accept responsibility for continuing education. The extent of the department's activity in this regard depends on available resources. As a minimum, the department should establish conferences in which clinical data, interesting pathology, and other fundamental material are presented and reviewed critically. Properly designed audit programs are useful in identifying needs for continuing education. In addition, obstetrician-gynecologists should take advantage of continuing educational programs sponsored by local, state, regional, and national organizations, by educational institutions, and by recognized recertification programs.

Physicians have an important role in planning and providing in-service education for nonmedical personnel.

GRADUATE MEDICAL EDUCATION

Physicians can integrate the information learned in medical school and develop diagnostic and therapeutic skills through graduate medical education. The quality of resident training depends on the standards of patient care maintained by the hospital and medical staff.

When a hospital provides graduate medical training, all patients should be considered part of the educational program. The educational value of this experience depends on department policies and on the attitudes of its members and their patients. To provide a meaningful learning experience, residents should participate in the pretreatment, treatment, and posttreatment evaluation of every patient to whom they are assigned. Residents should assume total care responsibility for their own patients under supervision of an attending staff physician. The resident should also be given increasing responsibilities involving patient care, surgical technique, and supervision of junior residents and medical students. The development of administrative abilities should not be neglected. With supervision, residents may also participate in the care of patients in the obstetrician-gynecologist's office, especially in the follow-up care of postoperative patients.

All attending physicians should be willing to participate in the graduate training program, providing continued supervision of the residents' activities.

COMMUNITY HEALTH

It is appropriate for the obstetrician-gynecologist to be involved in education, prevention, detection, and intervention programs designed to improve the general physical and mental health of community members. Through such involvement, the obstetrician-gynecologist can help to identify problems, establish priorities, and mobilize and coordinate all available community resources. A plan for regional perinatal care, for example, might be one outcome of such a community health improvement process.

Health service organizations concerned with primary care, maternal and infant care, and family planning require professional guidance if they are to develop and maintain high-quality service. The obstetrician-gynecologist, serving as a consultant or a direct provider of care within such an organization, should recognize that public programs must conform to specific regulations and guidelines. Obstetrician-gynecologists can render further community service as advisers to multidisciplinary staffs, e.g., outreach workers, social workers, nutritionists, and health care educators who provide patient services in community health facilities.

THE IMPAIRED PHYSICIAN

Practitioners should remain alert to behavioral changes that indicate an impairment in their colleagues. It is the responsibility of physicians to recognize a colleague's impairment, to assess the impairment, and to advise treatment or curtailment of practice.

Physicians allegedly impaired should be identified in a manner that protects their dignity and anonymity, and avoids unnecessary embarrassment. Every effort should be made to enlist their cooperation to acknowledge that a problem exists and to seek treatment.

The department head who becomes aware of deterioration in the performance of a staff member bears a special responsibility and should be capable of initiating an honest, nonjudgmental discussion of the situation with the physician. This discussion should include an evaluation of the impact that such a deterioration is having, and could have, on the physician's patients. The department director should develop a plan for the rehabilitation or reassignment of the physician in question. This plan may require the support of the physician's practice partners, other colleagues, the spouse, other family members, members of the clergy, counselors, and the physician's personal physician.

Appendix

Appendix 1

Bibliography

Accreditation Manual for Ambulatory Health Care (1985). Joint Commission on Accreditation of Hospitals (JCAH)*

Accreditation Manual for Hospitals (1985). JCAH*

Adolescent Perinatal Health, A Guidebook for Services (1985). ACOG.

Alternatives for Obstetric Design (1985). Ross Laboratories, Division of Abbott Laboratories, Columbus OH 43216

Ambulatory Health Care Standards Manual (1985). JCAH *

Assessment of Maternal Nutrition (1978). ACOG

Committee Statements, ACOG (Issued by ACOG Committees, these represent state-of-the-art opinions in obstetrics and gynecology. They are subject to change and are not to be considered ACOG policy. Complete listing of current titles is available from ACOG Resource Center.)
  Assessment of Fetal Maturity Prior to Repeat Cesarean Section and Elective Induction of Labor (1984)
  The Use of Cryotherapy in the Treatment of CIN (1984)
  Dystocia: Etiology, Diagnosis, and Management Guidelines (1983)
  Guidelines for Vaginal Delivery After Previous Cesarean Birth (1984)
  Human In Vitro Fertilization and Embryo Placement (1984)

A Design for Resident Education in Obstetrics and Gynecology (1981). Council on Resident Education in Obstetrics and Gynecology (CREOG)†

Educational Objectives for Residents in Obstetrics and Gynecology (1984). CREOG†

Family-Centered Maternity/Newborn Care in Hospitals (1978). Interprofessional Task Force Secretariat, ACOG

Guidelines for Childbirth Education (1981). The Nurses Association of the American College of Obstetricians and Gynecologists (NAACOG)‡

Guidelines For Perinatal Care, American Academy of Pediatrics (AAP)/ ACOG (1983). AAP Publications Department, P.O. Box 927, Elk Grove Village IL 60007

Guidelines on Pregnancy and Work (1977). ACOG

Gynecologic Health Record (1979). MILCOM, Division of Miller Communications, Inc., Norwalk CT 06856

Hollister Maternal and Newborn Record System (Revised 1981). Hollister, Inc. 2000 Hollister Drive, Libertyville IL 60048

How to Organize a Basic Study of the Infertile Couple (1981). The American Fertility Society, 1608 13th Avenue South, Suite 101, Birmingham AL 35256

Informed Consent for Invasive Therapy. The Assistant, Department of Professional Liability, ACOG

Obstetric-Gynecologic Nurse Practitioner (1984). NAACOG‡

Patient Education Pamphlets, ACOG (This series includes topics related to abortion, contraception, gynecologic problems, labor, delivery and postpartum care, physiology and sexuality, pregnancy, and women's health. Current listing of titles is available from ACOG Resource Center.)

Policy Statements, ACOG
Guidelines for Diagnostic X-Ray Examination of Fertile Women (1977)
Mammography (1979)
Periodic Cancer Screening in Women (1980)

Precis III: An Update in Obstetrics & Gynecology (1985). ACOG

Quality Assurance in Obstetrics and Gynecology (1981). ACOG

Resuscitation of the Newborn (1977). ACOG

Resuscitation of the Newborn (Film, 1977). Film and Video Service, P.O. Box 299, Wheaton IL 60189

Standards for Obstetric, Gynecologic, and Neonatal Nursing (1981). NAACOG‡

Technical Bulletins, ACOG (These provide timely information on the latest proven techniques of clinical practice in obstetrics and gynecology. Complete listing of current titles is available from the ACOG Resource Center.)
Anesthesia for Cesarean Section (1982)
Blood Component Therapy (1984)
Cancer of the Ovary (1983)
Carcinoma of the Endometrium (1984)
Carcinoma of the Vulva (1984)
Cervical Cytology: Evaluation and Management of Abnormalities (1984)
Diagnosis and Management of Invasive Cervical Carcinomas (1983)
Dysfunctional Uterine Bleeding (1982)
Epidemiology and Diagnosis of Breast Disease (1983)
Immunization During Pregnancy (1982)
Obstetric Anesthesia and Analgesia (1980)
Osteoporosis (1983)
Pregnancy, Work and Disability (1980)
Prenatal Detection of Neural Tube Defects (1982)
Prevention of Rho(D) Isoimmunization (1984)
Rubella—A Clinical Update (1981)

Toward Improving the Outcome of Pregnancy: Recommendations for the Regional Development of Maternal and Perinatal Health Services. Committee on Perinatal Health, The National Foundation–March of Dimes (1977)§

*Available from JCAH, Publications Department, 875 N. Michigan Ave., Chicago IL 60611

†Available from CREOG, 600 Maryland Ave., SW, Washington DC 20024

‡Available from NAACOG, 600 Maryland Ave., SW, Washington DC 20024

§Available through ACOG, 600 Maryland Ave., SW, Washington DC 20024

Appendix 2

OPERATIVE GYNECOLOGY:
Classification of Complications and Definitions

Unplanned Major Surgery is any surgical procedure for correcting a complication directly related to surgery performed either interoperatively or in the postoperative period during the same hospitalization.

Transfusion is any intraoperative or postoperative blood transfusion.

Febrile Morbidity is oral temperature 38.0 C on at least 2 postoperative days, excluding the first 24 hours after surgery.

Life-Threatening Event is any intraoperative or postoperative cardiac or respiratory arrest, cerebrovascular accident, myocardial infarction, pulmonary embolus, shock, or coagulopathy.

Rehospitalization is any readmission to a hospital within 6 weeks (42 days) of surgery because of a complaint or problem related to the primary operation.

Death is death or complication leading to death due to the operation or condition for which the operation was performed occurring within 6 weeks of surgery.

Appendix 3

The Role of the Obstetrician-Gynecologist in Women's Health Care

ACOG Statement of Policy as issued by the Executive Board, March 1979

Obstetrician-gynecologists are specialists who provide health care for women with particular reference to the female reproductive system. In addition to applying knowledge and skills to a specific organ system, they are involved in the care of the whole patient.

Obstetrician-gynecologists are the principal access and source of medical care and advice for many women throughout their adult lives, and may be their only regular medical contact. For other women they may serve solely as consultants. It is incumbent upon obstetrician-gynecologists that the patient clearly understands the scope of care to be offered and whether this will encompass responsibility for providing continuity for her personal health care. If continuity of care is not to be provided, the patient should be advised of the need for such care and offered assistance in locating an appropriate physician.

When providing continuity of care, obstetrician-gynecologists are responsible for collecting and regularly updating a defined data base, including history, physical examination, and appropriate laboratory procedures, for the patient population. Obstetrician-gynecologists will manage those problems relating to obstetrics and gynecology and whatever other disorders that lie within their capabilities. Problems outside the purview of obstetrician-gynecologists should be identified for the patient, who should then be offered guidance in obtaining appropriate care through referral. Follow-up of referred patients is essential for continuity of care and maintenance of a comprehensive data base.

Appendix 4

Ethical Considerations in the Practice of Obstetrics and Gynecology*

The medical profession has as its primary goal the health of the patients it serves through prevention, relief and cure of disease. In addition to this primary goal, the obstetrician-gynecologist has the specific objective of using special knowledge and skills to care for women in relation to the normal and abnormal structures and processes of human reproduction.

The American College of Obstetricians and Gynecologists was established to maintain a cooperating community of physicians to further the goal of the obstetrician-gynecologist. This involves the adherence by its Fellows to the social and ethical principles of honesty, loyalty, courtesy and respect for the rights of others—above all honesty. Fellows should support The American College of Obstetricians and Gynecologists as an organization dedicated to foster these principles and in addition should support legitimate educational, personal and professional interests of colleagues. No Fellow should use opportunities arising out of contact with patients, colleagues or the general public for self-aggrandizement or for demeaning the reputation of a colleague.

Fellows of The American College of Obstetricians and Gynecologists should seek to increase the effectiveness with which they pursue these principles by

1. Effective utilization of available knowledge and skills.
2. Support of and participation in medical education and research.
3. Provision for continuing education.
4. Advocacy of the utilization of specialized consultation and services when indicated and available.
5. Improvement, assistance in rehabilitation, or restriction of the impaired or incompetent Fellow.
6. Resistance to inappropriate interference in or restriction on the practice of high quality obstetrics and gynecology.
7. Support of institutional and organizational structures designed to achieve all of the above.

The Fellow who seeks to pursue a high ethical standard recognizes certain obligations to patients. For patients, the physician's ethical values of

---

* The Executive Board has approved these ethical considerations as information for Fellows and their patients. The College has adopted the AMA Code of Ethics as a policy.

honesty, courtesy, loyalty and respect for personal rights have special significance. These obligations include recognition of the patient's right

1. To be accorded respect and dignity without reference to age and sex or to marital, socioeconomic, ethnic, national, political, mental, physical or religious status.
2. To be free of exploitation by Fellows for social, sexual or personal gain.
3. To know the truth about her condition and treatment.
4. To full disclosure of financial factors involved in her treatment.
5. To make decisions regarding her own person, with access to relevant information on which to base such decisions.
6. To accept or to refuse treatment.
7. To freedom from coercion in such decision making.
8. To high quality medical care without regard to her status in life.
9. To the freedom to choose a physician and obtain additional consultation.
10. To know who will participate in her care.
11. To be fully informed and to decide whether to participate in or withdraw from medical research without jeopardizing the quality of her care.
12. Not to be neglected or discharged without opportunity to find other medical assistance.
13. To inviolable privacy except where this right is preempted by law.
14. To have an appropriate representative to exercise these rights when the patient herself is unable to do so.

The Fellow has certain rights in relation to patients, including the right

1. To refuse care, except in an emergency, to patients with whom no doctor-patient relationship has been established.
2. To discharge patients from care, providing adequate opportunity for other care has been extended.
3. To refuse to render treatment which is inconsistent with the Fellow's own moral code.
4. To retain control of clinical management as long as the physician-patient relationship remains intact.
5. To expect honest medically and socially relevant information from patients upon which to base care.
6. To receive reasonable compensation for services rendered.

There are certain rights and obligations that a Fellow owes to medical colleagues:

1. To adhere to the principle that ideally only one physician or physician group should be responsible for the general management of the patient's care at any one time, even when a designated portion of that care may be delegated to other professionals.
2. To remain, as the referring physician, responsible for the patient until the patient is either discharged or formally transferred.
3. To refuse the payment of any commission for referrals.
4. To give medical advice or treatment only to patients who are not now or no longer under the care of another physician except
   a. In an emergency where care shall be given until the patient's physician is available.
   b. When temporary coverage is provided by a Fellow for the patients of another physician.
   c. When consultation is formally requested by a patient or another physician.
5. To offer a fair and impartial review when rendering an opinion for legal purposes. An expert opinion should include all known facts and circumstances, and should not exclude any information in order to create a view favoring either plaintiff or defendant.

The Fellow should recognize certain obligations to the larger society:

1. To obey its laws, working through appropriate channels to change those which conflict with proper patient care.
2. To support those health programs and practices which contribute to the general public good.
3. To support those public policies which will help to achieve the above stated ethical principles.

Index

Abortion, 57, 60
  in ambulatory surgical facilities, 62–63
  pathologic evaluation in, 74
  timing of, 63
  for x-ray exposure, 85
Adolescent patients
  family planning services for, 56–57
  gynecologic care of, 58
  pregnancy in
    counseling for, 22
    nutritional requirements of, 19
Alcohol, use of, 16, 19
Ambulatory care
  facilities and equipment for, 24–26,
    64–65, 68–70
  of gynecologic patients, 51–70
  in free-standing and hospital-based sur-
    gical facilities, 61–62, 67–70
  administration of, 63–70
  medical services in, 53–59
  surgical services in, 60–63
  medical records of, 22–23, 63–64, 67–68
  of obstetric patients, 13–26
  administration of, 22–26
  services in, 15–22
  organization of, 3
  personnel for, 24, 64, 68
  in physician's office and outpatient clinic,
    60–61, 63–67
  quality assurance of, 23, 64, 68
Amniocentesis
  in ambulatory setting, 18
  for genetic evaluation, 19, 30
  in hospital care, 30
  for Rho(D) negative women, 18
Anesthesia
  for ambulatory surgery, 60, 61–62
  antepartum discussion of, 18
  in labor and delivery, 36–37
  and postpartum monitoring of patients,
    38
Antepartum care
  of adolescents, 21–22
  ambulatory, 15–26

Antepartum care *(continued)*
  frequency of visits for, 17–18
  health and childbirth education in, 20
  history in, 16
  in hospitals, 30–31
  initial evaluation in, 15–17, 31
  laboratory tests in, 16
  monitoring procedures in, 18, 30
  occupational considerations in, 21
  physical examination in, 16, 18
  psychosocial services in, 21
  risk assessment of, 17
  screening for genetic disorders in, 18–19
Antibody screening
  antepartum, 16, 18
  for gynecologic patients, 75
Apgar score, 38

Birth defects, *see* Genetic disorders
Birthing room
  facilities and equipment for, 48–49
  recovery care in, 38
  standards of care of, 35–36
Blood tests
  antepartum, 16, 18, 30, 33
  capabilities in hospitals of, 30
  for gynecologic patients, on admission,
    15
Breast
  disease of, 55–56
  Self-examination of, 53, 55
Breast-feeding, 20, 39
  and maternal nutritional requirements,
    20

Caloric requirements
  of breast-feeding, 20
  of pregnancy, 20
Cancer
  of breast, 55–56
  chemotherapy for, 73
  hospital care of, 73, 74